Endovascular Interventions

Endovascular Interventions

A Step-by-Step Approach

Edited by

Jose M. Wiley, MD, MPH
Sidney W. and Marilyn S. Lassen Chair of Cardiovascular Medicine
Professor of Medicine
Chief, Section of Cardiology
John W. Deming Department of Medicine
Tulane University School of Medicine
New Orleans, LA, USA

Cristina Sanina, MD
Interventional Cardiology Fellow
Division of Cardiology
Department of Medicine
Beth Israel Deaconess Medical Center
Harvard Medical School
Boston, MA, USA

George D. Dangas, MD, PhD
Professor of Medicine
Director of Cardiovascular Innovations
The Zena and Michael A. Weiner Cardiovascular Institute
Icahn School of Medicine at Mount Sinai
New York, NY, USA

Prakash Krishnan, MD
Professor of Medicine
Director of Endovascular Services
The Zena and Michael A. Weiner Cardiovascular Institute
Icahn School of Medicine at Mount Sinai
New York, NY, USA

WILEY Blackwell

The right of Jose M. Wiley, Cristina Sanina, George D. Dangas, and Prakash Krishnan to be identified as the authors of the editorial material in this work has been asserted in accordance with law.

Registered Offices
John Wiley & Sons, Inc., 111 River Street, Hoboken, NJ 07030, USA
John Wiley & Sons Ltd, The Atrium, Southern Gate, Chichester, West Sussex, PO19 8SQ, UK

For details of our global editorial offices, customer services, and more information about Wiley products visit us at www.wiley.com.

Wiley also publishes its books in a variety of electronic formats and by print-on-demand. Some content that appears in standard print versions of this book may not be available in other formats.

Library of Congress Cataloging-in-Publication Data
Names: Wiley, Jose M., author. | Sanina, Cristina, author. | Dangas, George
  D., author. | Krishnan, Prakash, author.
Title: Endovascular interventions: a step-by-step approach / Jose M. Wiley,
  Cristina Sanina, George D. Dangas, Prakash Krishnan.
Description: Hoboken, NJ : Wiley-Blackwell, 2023. | Includes
  bibliographical references and index.
Identifiers: LCCN 2023012153 (print) | LCCN 2023012154 (ebook) |
  ISBN 9781119467786 (paperback) | ISBN 9781119467847 (adobe pdf) |
  ISBN 9781119467861 (epub)
Subjects: MESH: Endovascular Interventions.
Classification: LCC RD598.5 (print) | LCC RD598.5 (ebook) | NLM WG 170 |
  DDC 617.4/13–dc23/eng/20230531
LC record available at https://lccn.loc.gov/2023012153
LC ebook record available at https://lccn.loc.gov/2023012154

Cover Design: Wiley
Cover Image: © Cristina Sanina

Set in 9.5/12.5pt STIXTwoText by Straive, Pondicherry, India
Printed in Singapore
M084763_040723

Contents

List of Contributors

Tyrone J. Collins, MD
Department of Cardiovascular
Diseases, John Ochsner Heart &
Vascular Institute, The Ochsner
Clinical School, University of
Queensland School of Medicine
New Orleans, LA, USA

Saadat Shariff, MD
Department of Cardiothoracic &
Vascular Surgery (Vascular Surgery)
Albert Einstein College of Medicine-
Montefiore Medical Center
Bronx, NY, USA

Isabella Alviz, MD
Department of Medicine, Albert
Einstein College of Medicine-
Montefiore Medical Center
Bronx, NY, USA

Cornelia Rivera, MD
Department of Medicine, Albert
Einstein College of Medicine-
Montefiore Medical Center
Bronx, NY, USA

Michelle Cortorreal, MD
Department of Medicine, Albert
Einstein College of Medicine-
Montefiore Medical Center
Bronx, NY, USA

James S. Jenkins, MD
Department of Cardiovascular
Diseases, John Ochsner Heart &
Vascular Institute, The Ochsner
Clinical School, University of
Queensland School of Medicine
New Orleans, LA, USA

Tamunoinemi Bob-Manuel, MD
Department of Cardiovascular
Diseases, John Ochsner Heart &
Vascular Institute, The Ochsner
Clinical School, University of
Queensland School of Medicine
New Orleans, LA, USA

Aksim G. Rivera, MD
Department of Surgery (Vascular
Surgery), Albert Einstein College
of Medicine-Jacobi Medical Center
Bronx, NY, USA

Patricia Yau, MD
Department of Surgery (Vascular
Surgery), Albert Einstein College
of Medicine-Jacobi Medical Center
Bronx, NY, USA

John Denesopolis, MD
Department of Surgery (Vascular
Surgery), Albert Einstein College
of Medicine-Jacobi Medical Center
Bronx, NY, USA

John Futchko, MD
Department of Surgery (Vascular
Surgery), Albert Einstein College
of Medicine-Jacobi Medical Center
Bronx, NY, USA

Katie MacCallum, MD
Department of Surgery (Vascular
Surgery), Albert Einstein College
of Medicine-Jacobi Medical Center
Bronx, NY, USA

Mohammad Hashim Mustehsan, MD
Division of Cardiology, Albert Einstein
College of Medicine-Montefiore
Medical Center, Bronx, NY, USA

Jose D. Tafur, MD
Department of Cardiovascular
Diseases, John Ochsner Heart &
Vascular Institute, The Ochsner
Clinical School, University of
Queensland School of Medicine
New Orleans, LA, USA

Cristina Sanina, MD
Division of Cardiology
Department of Medicine
Beth Israel Deaconess Medical Center
Harvard Medical School
Boston, MA, USA

David A. Hirschl, MD
Department of Radiology, Albert
Einstein College of Medicine-
Montefiore Medical Center
Bronx, NY, USA

Michael S. Segal, DO
Department of General Surgery
Wyckoff Heights Medical Center
Brooklyn, NY, USA

Sameh Elrabie, DO
Department of General Surgery
Wyckoff Heights Medical Center
Brooklyn, NY, USA

Rajesh K. Malik, MD
Division of Vascular Surgery
Wyckoff Heights Medical Center
Brooklyn, NY, USA

Sahil A. Parikh, MD
Division of Cardiovascular Diseases
Columbia University Irving Medical
Center, New York, NY, USA

Joseph J. Ingrassia, MD
Division of Cardiovascular Diseases
Columbia University Irving Medical
Center, New York, NY, USA

Matthew T. Finn, MD
Division of Cardiovascular Diseases
Columbia University Irving Medical
Center, New York, NY, USA

Raman Sharma, MD
Division of Cardiology, The Zena and
Michael A. Weiner Cardiovascular
Institute, Icahn School of Medicine at
Mount Sinai, New York, NY, USA

Prakash Krishnan, MD
Division of Cardiology, The Zena and
Michael A. Weiner Cardiovascular
Institute, Icahn School of Medicine at
Mount Sinai, New York, NY, USA

Roberto Cerrud-Rodriguez, MD
Division of Cardiology, Albert Einstein
College of Medicine-Montefiore
Medical Center, Bronx, NY, USA

Shunsuke Aoi, MD
Division of Cardiology, Albert Einstein
College of Medicine-Montefiore
Medical Center, Bronx, NY, USA

Amit M. Kakkar, MD
Division of Cardiology, Albert Einstein
College of Medicine-Jacobi Medical
Center, Bronx, NY, USA

Ehrin J. Armstrong, MD
University of Colorado School of
Medicine-Rocky Mountain Regional
VA Medical Center, CO, USA

Rory Brinker, MD
University of Colorado School of
Medicine-Rocky Mountain Regional
VA Medical Center, CO, USA

Manaf Assafin, MD
Division of Cardiology, Albert Einstein
College of Medicine-Montefiore
Medical Center, Bronx, NY, USA

Miguel Alvarez-Villela, MD
Division of Cardiology, Albert Einstein
College of Medicine-Montefiore
Medical Center, Bronx, NY, USA

Robert Pyo, MD
Division of Cardiology, Renaissance
School of Medicine at Stony Brook
University, NY, USA

Pedro Cox-Alomar, MD
Division of Cardiology, Louisiana
State University School of Medicine
New Orleans, LA, USA

Vishal Kapur, MD
Division of Cardiology, The Zena and
Michael A. Weiner Cardiovascular
Institute, Icahn School of Medicine at
Mount Sinai, New York, NY, USA

Sagar Goyal, MD
Division of Cardiology, The Zena and
Michael A. Weiner Cardiovascular
Institute, Icahn School of Medicine at
Mount Sinai, New York, NY, USA

Asma Khaliq, MD
Department of Cardiology, Lenox
Hill Heart & Vascular Institute
Donald and Barbara Zucker School of
Medicine at Hofstra/Northwell Health
New York, NY, USA

Sandrine Labrune, MD
Department of Cardiology, Lenox
Hill Heart & Vascular Institute
Donald and Barbara Zucker School of
Medicine at Hofstra/Northwell Health
New York, NY, USA

Seth I. Sokol, MD
Division of Cardiovascular
Diseases, Albert Einstein College
of Medicine-Jacobi Medical Center
Bronx, NY, USA

Wissam A. Jaber, MD
Division of Cardiology, Emory
University Hospital, Atlanta, GA, USA

Yosef Golowa, MD
Department of Radiology, Albert
Einstein College of Medicine-
Montefiore Medical Center
Bronx, NY, USA

Juan Terre, MD
Division of Cardiology, Albert Einstein
College of Medicine-Montefiore
Medical Center, Bronx, NY, USA

Nelson Chavarria, MD, MSc
Division of Cardiology, Albert Einstein
College of Medicine-Montefiore
Medical Center, Bronx, NY, USA

Jose M. Wiley, MD, MPH
Section of Cardiology
John W. Deming Department of
Medicine
Tulane University School of Medicine
New Orleans, LA, USA

George D. Dangas, MD, PhD
Division of Cardiology, The Zena and
Michael A. Weiner Cardiovascular
Institute, Icahn School of Medicine at
Mount Sinai, New York, NY, USA

1

Innominate & Carotid Artery Intervention in High-Risk Patients

Tyrone J. Collins

Department of Cardiovascular Diseases, John Ochsner Heart & Vascular Institute, The Ochsner Clinical School, University of Queensland School of Medicine, New Orleans, LA, USA

Introduction

Revascularization of supra-aortic arterial disease (complicated peripheral artery disease) is usually elective and prophylactic to prevent initial or recurrent ischemic events. Surgical revascularization was once considered the treatment of choice [1]. Successful reports of percutaneous transluminal angioplasty (PTA) and stenting introduced endovascular treatment as an equal or possibly better than surgery option [2]. Each patient is unique, and the risk is multifactorial with both demographic and anatomic risk factors.

Several "high-risk" features are generally considered when treating carotid artery disease in these patients [3] (Table 1.1). Some of these features are also risk factors for innominate intervention.

The level of stenosis and/or occlusion, vessel tortuosity, amount of calcification, presence or absence of thrombus, concomitant vascular abnormalities, and comorbid conditions will also affect the risk with revascularization of the other supra-aortic vessels.

Although some authors may consider endovascular therapy the treatment of choice for innominate atherosclerotic disease, surgical therapy has been shown to be safe and effective [4]. During a period of almost 20 years from 1974 to 1993, Kieffer et al. revascularized surgically 148 patients with acceptable rates of complications, late mortality, long-term patency, freedom from neurologic events, and reoperation [4].

Endovascular Interventions: A Step-by-Step Approach, First Edition. Edited by Jose M. Wiley, Cristina Sanina, George D. Dangas, and Prakash Krishnan.

Table 1.1   High-risk features reported in the literature.

1) CAS in females
2) CAS in octogenarians
3) CAS with type II, type III, or bovine arch
4) Tortuous common carotid artery, angulated ICA, and/or distal ICA
5) Long lesions ≥15 mm
6) Ostial-centered lesions
7) Calcified arch and/or heavily calcified lesion
8) High-grade stenosis
9) Contralateral carotid occlusion
10) Presence of vertebral artery occlusion and/or stenosis
11) Patient with CKD

Innominate Interventions in High-Risk Patients

Catheter-based Therapy for An Innominate (Brachiocephalic) Stenosis

Step 1. Identification of the level of stenosis is the initial step. Computed tomography angiography (CTA) can be useful prior to an invasive procedure. This can allow for planning the interventional strategy and considering alternative forms of treatment. Additionally, CTA can be used to size the reference vessels.

When considering the choice of arterial access remember that catheter size is limited with radial access and the need to cross the stenosis is usually necessary from the radial or brachial approach. If intervention is planned, injections are against the direction of blood flow when working from the arm approach. I prefer the femoral approach to innominate stenoses.

Invasive angiography can be done with digital and/or subtraction angiography. A pigtail catheter is positioned in the ascending aorta proximal to the origin of the innominate artery. The angiography is performed in the 30° left anterior oblique (LAO) projection. Selective angiography is done with a Judkins right diagnostic catheter or guiding catheter (Figure 1.1a,b). Other diagnostic catheters can be used for selective angiography. The "working view" is the angulation that allows for delineation of the stenosis, any adjacent branches, and the ostium of the innominate. Road mapping may be useful but also take advantage of any vascular calcification as a point of reference.

Step 2. After the decision to intervene and baseline angiography has been performed, the innominate is engaged with an 8 Fr guide catheter. A different approach is to use a diagnostic catheter to engage the innominate artery, cross the stenosis with the appropriate wire, and introduce a 6 Fr sheath over the wire to the

(a)   (b)

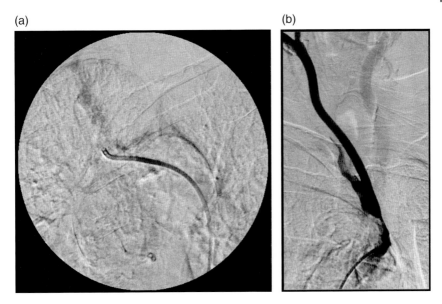

Figure 1.1 (a) Heavily calcified aorta and supra-aortic vessels. (b) Baseline innominate artery selective angiogram.

ostium of the innominate. Anticoagulation to achieve an activated clotting time (ACT) > 250 s is administered. Depending on the available balloons and stents, the appropriate wire (0.014–0.035 in.) is steered across the stenosis. The tip of the wire is passed into the subclavian artery. Wire tip can also be placed in the common or external carotid artery. Innominate artery PTA and stenting is usually performed without utilizing a distal embolic protection device (EPD). If you choose to use EPD, the necessary wire or filter can be positioned in the internal carotid artery. Horesh reported a case of innominate stenting with a covered stent and distal protection [5]. He emphasized the need to individualize patients and consider using embolic protection in high-risk patients. Hybrid procedures have been performed using balloon occlusion to trap embolic debris.

Step 3. Predilatation with a balloon is performed. The initial balloon is usually undersized but gives an idea of the ability to distend the lesion (Figure 1.2). The Shockwave Lithoplasty System (Medical Inc.) has been used to successfully treat severely calcified innominate stenosis prior to stenting [6]. This system has also been used in a hybrid operation [7]. Use the balloon inflation to help decide on stent sizing (diameter and length).

Step 4. Stent implantation is done after ensuring the correct position of the delivery system (Figure 1.3). If necessary, magnify the image to demonstrate the stent is appropriately placed. Remember, an undersized stent can be implanted so that

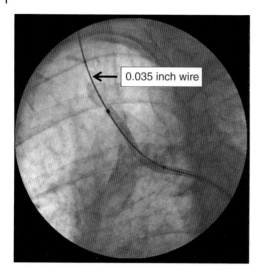

Figure 1.2 Predilatation with undersized balloon.

0.035 inch wire

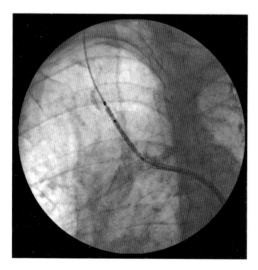

Figure 1.3 Stent in position at ostium of innominate.

the delivery sheath or catheter does not have to be "upsized." A larger balloon (Figure 1.4) can subsequently be employed to adequately expand the stent without changing the sheath or catheter.

Step 5. Assessment of the poststent result is performed to determine stent apposition and size (Figure 1.5). If necessary, the stent can be postdilated with a larger balloon.

Step 6. After hemostasis the patient is usually monitored overnight and discharged the following day. Dual antiplatelet therapy is maintained for at least one month if there are no contraindications.

Figure 1.4 Larger balloon inflation.

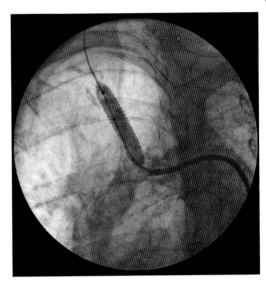

Figure 1.5 Final angiogram.

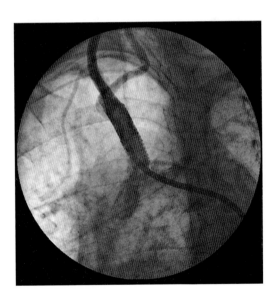

Carotid Artery Intervention in High-Risk Patients

Endovascular Treatment of A Carotid Stenosis

Left common carotid artery stenoses are treated endovascularly similarly to innominate artery stenoses. Distal embolic protection is not used routinely. There are endovascular, hybrid, and surgical alternatives.

Transcarotid artery revascularization (TCAR) offers alternative to both carotid endarterectomy (CEA) and carotid artery stenting (CAS) which are done via a transfemoral approach.

CAS can be performed with distal embolic protection and/or flow reversal. Distal embolic protection is the most commonly used choice. It is readily available and technically easier to deploy. However, it is not the best choice for tortuous common and/or internal carotid arteries, heavily calcified vessels, and "string signs." Distal protection devices require crossing the diseased segment without protection compared to proximal protection where this is not necessary. Additionally, if anatomy warrants, CEA can be the treatment of choice.

Catheter-based Therapy for Carotid Stenosis

Step 1. Arterial access is obtained for distal embolic protection and flow reversal cases. Distal EPD can be done via femoral, radial, or brachial access. Flow reversal, because of the larger diameter sheath required, is performed via the femoral artery route. Access is obtained with ultrasound guidance or using anatomic landmarks. Femoral angiography is usually performed at the initiation of the case to document the appropriateness of the access and to plan for use of a closure device (Figure 1.6).

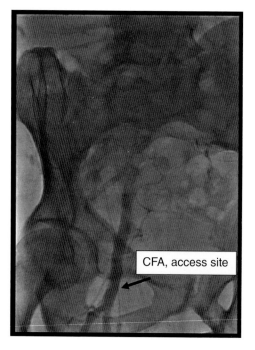

Figure 1.6 Femoral artery access.

CFA, access site

Figure 1.7 Baseline selective angiography with reference object.

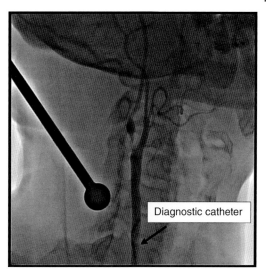

Diagnostic catheter

Step 2. Selective carotid angiography (Figure 1.7) of the culprit vessel is performed with a diagnostic catheter. The best angle to visualize the lesion is chosen. Quantitative angiography is done. This can be with a reference object placed at the level of the lesion or with online software. Of note, angiography of all the arch and intracranial vessels is performed prior to intervention. This can be done during the CAS procedure or at an earlier date. Other imaging modalities (CTA or MRI) can be done prior to the CAS. Imaging of the intracranial circulation is necessary in the event that the rare occurrence of neurorescue is needed and it is necessary to document the baseline anatomy.

Step 3. Heparin is administered to achieve an ACT greater than 250 s. A sheath, guide catheter, or neuroprotection device is exchanged over a stiff wire (exchange length 0.035 in. Amplatz wire). The tip is placed in the common carotid artery. During the exchange procedure, the tip of the wire is positioned in the common carotid or external carotid artery. For the flow reversal case, it is necessary to place the stiff wire in the external carotid artery (ECA) through the diagnostic catheter (Figure 1.8) before the exchange procedure.

Step 4. This is where the proximal and distal protection significantly differ. With distal protection, a device is passed through the lesion into the internal carotid artery (Figure 1.9). The EPD is deployed. Balloon predilatation (Figures 1.10) is usually done with a smaller than the reference vessel sized balloon (generally 2.5–3 mm). A stent is deployed (Figure 1.11) and usually postdilatation is skipped. Completion angiography is done (Figure 1.12) along with the intracranial images. Hemostasis can be obtained with a closure device of choice. Generally, these patients are observed in the hospital overnight.

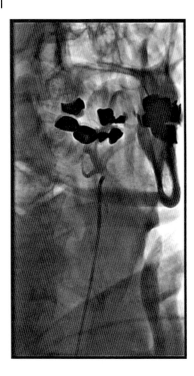

Figure 1.8 Angiogram through a diagnostic catheter in the external carotid artery before exchange.

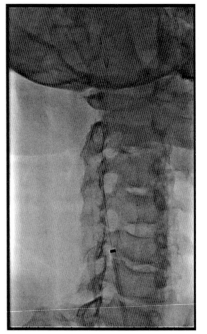

Figure 1.9 EPD positioned in the internal carotid artery.

Figure 1.10 Predilatation with distal embolic protection.

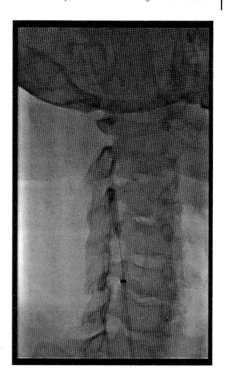

Figure 1.11 Retrieval of the EPD.

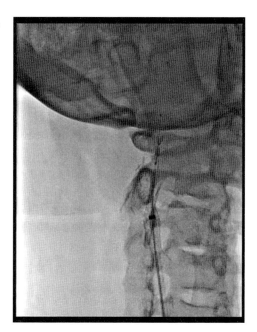

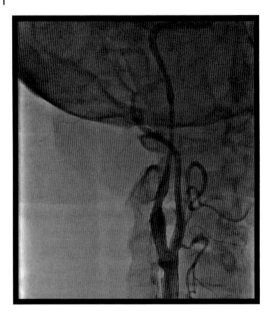

Figure 1.12 Final angiogram after stenting.

When flow reversal is used, it follows the instructions for use with the Medtronic Mo.Ma device. The ECA balloon is inflated in the proximal segment (Figure 1.13). The common carotid balloon is inflated and the stenting is performed (Figures 1.14–1.16) with flow reversal at the end of the procedure prior to reestablishing antegrade flow. Operator should have all equipment ready to insert. I encourage "loading" the balloon and wire in the catheter before starting the proximal occlusion to minimize the occlusion time. Completion angiography, hemostasis, and postoperative care are as above with distal embolic protection.

Conclusions

The operator must carefully consider if revascularization is indicated in the patient with supra-aortic atherosclerosis. Revascularization is usually performed prophylactically to prevent ischemic events. The risk must be considered compared to the potential benefits. Knowledge of alternative revascularization strategies is paramount before undertaking these procedures.

Figure 1.13 Mo.Ma device with ECA balloon inflated.

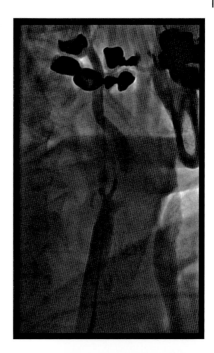

Figure 1.14 Stent and postdilatation.

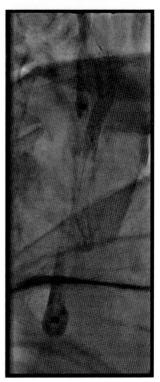

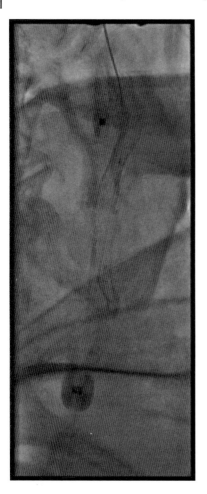

Figure 1.15 ECA balloon deflated with proximal balloon inflated.

Figure 1.16 Final angiogram.

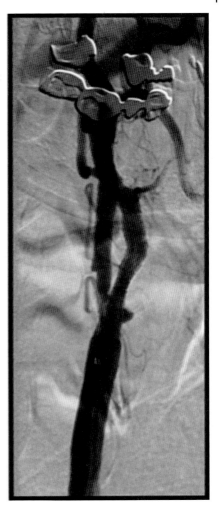

References

1 Sullivan, T.M., Gray, B.H., Bacharach, J.M. et al. (1998). Angioplasty and primary stenting of the subclavian, innominate and common carotid arteries in 83 patients. *J. Vasc. Surg.* 28: 1059–1065.

2 Motarjeme, A. (1996). Percutaneous transluminal angioplasty of supra-aortic vessels. *J. Endovasc. Surg.* 3: 171–181.

3 Elewa, M.K. (2019). *Carotid Artery Stenting in High-Risk Patients for Stenting, Carotid Artery - Gender and Health* (ed. R. Rezzani and L.F. Rodella). IntechOpen https://doi.org/10.5772/intechopen.82019.

4 Kieffer, E., Sabatier, J., Koskas, F., and Bahnini, A. (1995). Atherosclerotic innominate artery occlusive disease: early and long-term results of surgical reconstruction. *J. Vasc. Surg.* 21: 326–337.

5 Horesh, L. (2010). Endovascular management of an embolizing innominate artery stenosis: Evaluation of distal protection devices and covered stents. *Endovascular Today* 36–40.

6 Tripolino, C., Grillo, P., Tassone, E.J. et al. (2019). A case of critical calcified innominate artery stenosis successfully treated with the Shockwave Lithoplasty. *Clin. Med. Insights Case Rep.* 12: 1–3.

7 Mordasini, P., Gralla, J., Do, D.D. et al. (2011). Stenting of symptomatic high-grade innominate artery stenosis: technique and follow-up. *AJNR Am. J. Neuroradiol.* 32: 1726–1731.

2

Subclavian Artery Intervention

Catheter-Based Therapy

Saadat Shariff[1], Isabella Alviz[2], Cornelia Rivera[3],
Michelle Cortorreal[3], and Tyrone J. Collins[4]

[1] Department of Cardiothoracic & Vascular Surgery (Vascular Surgery), Albert Einstein College of Medicine-Montefiore Medical Center, Bronx, NY, USA
[2] Department of Medicine, Albert Einstein College of Medicine-Montefiore Medical Center, Bronx, NY, USA
[3] Department of Medicine, Albert Einstein College of Medicine-Montefiore Medical Center, Bronx, NY, USA
[4] Department of Cardiovascular Diseases, John Ochsner Heart & Vascular Institute, University of Queensland School of Medicine, New Orleans, LA, USA

Introduction

The occurrence of subclavian artery (SA) stenosis or occlusion is low compared to lower extremity disease with a prevalence of approximately 2–3% in the general population [1, 2]. Atherosclerosis is the most common cause for hemodynamically significant lesions with arteritis, and aneurysmal disease being less common. The left SA is more commonly affected than the right side, with a slight male to female predominance. Most patients are asymptomatic, and treatment is generally recommended for symptomatic patients. Symptoms that warrant intervention include vertebrobasilar insufficiency, arm claudication, and transient ischemic attacks. Less commonly, interventions are performed for protection of an arteriovenous fistula or prevention of coronary steal syndrome in patients with prior internal mammary coronary bypass surgery. Endovascular intervention for SA stenosis became the first line of treatment.

Endovascular Interventions: A Step-by-Step Approach, First Edition. Edited by Jose M. Wiley, Cristina Sanina, George D. Dangas, and Prakash Krishnan.
© 2023 John Wiley & Sons Ltd. Published 2023 by John Wiley & Sons Ltd.

Endovascular Versus Open Surgical Revascularization

Optimal treatment for SA occlusive disease has been controversial ever since the introduction of endovascular interventions [3]. Percutaneous balloon angioplasty of SA stenosis was first described in 1980 by Bachman and Kim. Since then, several studies have compared the durability of endovascular repair to the conventional open surgical repair. Open surgical repair has better long-term patency compared to endovascular repair, 96% compared to 70% at five years, respectively [4, 5]. AbuRahma et al. showed that technical success rate was similar in both the groups, the open repair group had better long-term patency and recurrence of symptoms compared to the endovascular group [4]. However, with the advancements in endovascular techniques in the last three decades, endovascular repair has become the first choice for SA revascularization. Several studies have shown primary patency rates of 77–93% at one year and 72–93% at three to eight years, respectively [6–9]. The technical success of treating SA lesions varies dramatically for stenosis compared to occlusions. SA occlusions especially ostial lesions are more difficult to treat compared to stenosis. Some have reported technical success ranging from 50 to 100% for occlusions compared to stenosis ranging from 91 to 100%. Jahic et al. reported 100% success rate with SA stenosis and only 55.5% success in total occlusions, respectively [10].

Endovascular Revascularization Techniques

Step 1. Transfemoral approach is generally preferred and initiated using the Seldinger technique; however, brachial and combined femoral-brachial access may also be used. Once access is achieved, a short or long introduction sheath is placed and a nonselective aortic arch angiogram in the left anterior oblique (LAO) position is performed using a soft multi-hole catheter (pigtail catheter, etc.), which minimizes the risk of aortic dissection during contrast injection. Contrast material (30–40 ml) may be delivered using auto-injection at a rate of 15–20 ml/s over 2–3 s (0.3–0.5 s rate of rise and 900 psi). Hand injection (5–10 ml) may be used for selective angiography with a Judkins Right 4 (JR4), multipurpose (MPA), or Berenstein catheter. Catheter selection is mainly guided by aortic arch anatomy. For instance, for a type I aortic arch, the use of a JR4 catheter is appropriate. For a type II arch, a Vitek (VTK) or Headhunter-1 (H-1) catheter is recommended, whereas a Simmons 1 or 2 (SIMS) is typically used for a type III arch. In most cases, the use of two orthogonal oblique views is sufficient for proper visualization. The use of digital subtraction angiography (DSA) provides enhanced delineation of the vasculature. The brachiocephalic bifurcation, right SA origin, proximal left vertebral artery, and left internal mammary artery (IMA) origin are best viewed in the right anterior oblique (RAO) views. The right vertebral artery and right IMA are best seen in the LAO view.

Step 2. Once a guide is placed proximal to the lesion, the lesion is carefully crossed with a guide wire and percutaneous transluminal angioplasty (PTAS) is performed. The main issue with lone PTAS is the need for reintervention in restenosis, which has been reported to be as high as 21% at three years follow-up. Importantly, using an undersized balloon (~70% of the vessel diameter) helps reducing the risk of dissection during predilatation. Technical success in stenting is extremely high (98%) (Figure 2.1a–c) [11]. In the largest case series to date with 170 patients, 177 stents were placed (94% subclavian and 6% innominate arteries) without any procedural deaths and very low major complication rates (0.6%). Primary and secondary patency rates at five years were reported at 83 and 98%, respectively. A large meta-analysis of 35 noncomparative studies involving 1726 patients compared PTAS and stent placement for SA stenosis and confirmed significantly higher technical success rates in the stent group compared to the PTAS

(a)

(c)

(b)

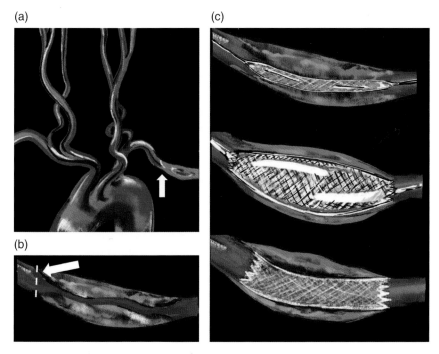

Figure 2.1 Left-sided subclavian stenosis. (a) and (b) arrows show initiation of stenotic region. (c) Careful crossing of the stenosis over a guide wire followed by PTAS and successful stent deployment. *Source:* Artist credit: Cristina Sanina.

(a)   (b)   (c)   (d)

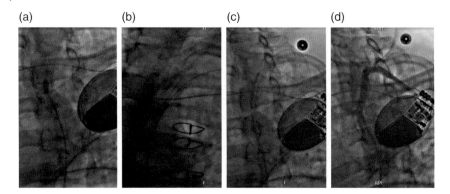

Figure 2.2 (a) Catheter engaged in ostium left subclavian artery and previous stent with dye injection showing complete occlusion. (b) Attempts at antegrade advancement of the guide wire through the occlusion were unsuccessful. This picture shows successful guide wire advanced across the occlusion from a retrograde approach. (c) New stent positioned across the occlusion. (d) Complete restoration of flow to the subclavian and LIMA after stent deployment.

group (92.8 vs. 86.8%, p = 0.007) [12]. Interestingly, both long-term primary patency rates and symptom resolution rates were not significantly different between the two groups. Although very uncommon, in-stent thrombosis and restenosis occurrence may be technically challenging, but amenable to redilatation. Both antegrade (via radial or brachial artery access) approaches may be helpful in guide wire advancement across the occlusion. Once this is accomplished, balloon angioplasty or restenting can be done in the usual fashion for flow restoration (Figure 2.2). For stenosis proximal to the vertebral artery and IMA, balloon expandable stents are used for more accurate placement. For stenosis distal to the vertebral artery and IMA, self-expanding stents are used, and these provide more flexibility and deformability, but less placement accuracy. Typical sizes for the SA range from 6 to 8 mm in diameter. Complications of endovascular intervention include, but are not limited to, access site hematomas, dissection, perforation, rupture, distal embolization, stroke, transient ischemic attack (TIA) and arterial thrombosis [13].

Conclusion

Open surgical revascularization has been the gold standard for SA lesions but with the advancements in endovascular surgery in the last few decades, it was become the first line of treatment. A step-by-step approach is necessary in order to standardize the procedure and avoid complications.

References

1 Shadman, R., Criqui, M.H., Bundens, W.P. et al. (2004). Subclavian artery stenosis: prevalence, risk factors, and association with cardiovascular diseases. *J. Am. Coll. Cardiol.* 44: 618–623.

2 Ochoa, V.M. and Yeghiazarians, Y. (2011). Subclavian artery stenosis: a review for the vascular medicine practitioner. *Vasc. Med.* 16: 29–34.

3 Bachman, D.M. and Kim, R.M. (1980). Transluminal dilatation for subclavian steal syndrome. *AJR Am. J. Roentgenol.* 135: 995–996.

4 AbuRahma, A.F., Bates, M.C., Stone, P.A. et al. (2007). Angioplasty and stenting versus carotid-subclavian bypass for the treatment of isolated subclavian artery disease. *J. Endovasc. Ther.* 14: 698–704.

5 Palchik, E., Bakken, A.M., Wolford, H.Y. et al. (2008). Subclavian artery revascularization: an outcome analysis based on mode of therapy and presenting symptoms. *Ann. Vasc. Surg.* 22: 70–78.

6 Przewlocki, T., Kablak-Ziembicka, A., Pieniazek, P. et al. (2006). Determinants of immediate and long-term results of subclavian and innominate artery angioplasty. *Catheter. Cardiovasc. Interv.* 67: 519–526.

7 Sixt, S., Rastan, A., Schwarzwalder, U. et al. (2009). Results after balloon angioplasty or stenting of atherosclerotic subclavian artery obstruction. *Catheter. Cardiovasc. Interv.* 73: 395–403.

8 Brountzos, E.N., Petersen, B., Binkert, C. et al. (2004). Primary stenting of subclavian and innominate artery occlusive disease: a single center's experience. *Cardiovasc. Intervent. Radiol.* 27: 616–623.

9 Benhammamia, M., Mazzaccaro, D., Ben Mrad, M. et al. (2020). Endovascular and surgical management of subclavian artery occlusive disease: early and long-term outcomes. *Ann. Vasc. Surg.* 66: 462–469.

10 Jahic, E., Avdagic, H., Iveljic, I., and Krdzalic, K. (2019). Percutaneous transluminal angioplasty of subclavian artery lesions. *Med. Arch.* 73 (1): 28–31.

11 Patel, S.N., White, C.J., Collins, T.J. et al. (2008). Catheter-based treatment of the subclavian and innominate arteries. *Catheter. Cardiovasc. Interv.* 71: 963–968.

12 Ahmed, A.T., Mohammed, K., Chehab, M. et al. (2016). Comparing percutaneous transluminal angioplasty and stent placement for treatment of subclavian arterial occlusive disease: a systematic review and meta-analysis. *Cardiovasc. Intervent. Radiol.* 39: 652–667.

13 Henry, M., Amor, M., Henry, I. et al. (1999). Percutaneous transluminal angioplasty of the subclavian arteries. *J. Endovasc. Surg.* 6: 33–41.

3

Vertebral Artery Intervention

Catheter-Based Therapy

Tamunoinemi Bob-Manuel and James S. Jenkins

Department of Cardiovascular Diseases, John Ochsner Heart & Vascular Institute, The Ochsner Clinical School, University of Queensland School of Medicine, New Orleans, LA, USA

Introduction

Endovascular treatment of the ostial and proximal portion of the vertebral artery is a safe and effective technique for alleviating symptoms and improving cerebral blood flow to the posterior circulation [1–3]. Vertebral artery angioplasty can be performed with high technical and clinical success rates, low complication rates, and durable long-term results [4]. Although restenosis rates vary widely, the durability of vertebral artery angioplasty is evidenced by low restenosis rates in several large series reported in the literature using multiple treatment options, including balloon angioplasty alone, bare-metal stents, and drug-coated stents [5]. Endovascular stenting of vertebral artery atherosclerotic disease in patients who fail medical therapy should be considered first-line therapy despite the absence of randomized trials demonstrating superiority of endovascular therapy. Defining the anatomy of the vertebral artery, including proximal inflow and collateral pathways, is necessary to determine the appropriate vessel that provides the best revascularization to the posterior circulation [6]. The use of coronary angioplasty equipment and proper guide selection will allow safe and effective treatment of complex vertebral lesions. Although off-label, EPD should be considered to prevent distal embolic complications if vertebral artery anatomy is suitable.

Endovascular treatment of the vertebral artery is a less invasive alternative than open surgery and should become the preferred therapy for symptomatic vertebral artery atherosclerotic obstructive disease not responsive to medical therapy.

Endovascular Interventions: A Step-by-Step Approach, First Edition. Edited by Jose M. Wiley, Cristina Sanina, George D. Dangas, and Prakash Krishnan.
© 2023 John Wiley & Sons Ltd. Published 2023 by John Wiley & Sons Ltd.

Preprocedural Considerations

All patients should be loaded with aspirin (325 mg) and an antiplatelet preferably clopidogrel (300–600 mg) at least one day prior to the procedure. Minimal or no sedation should be used during the procedure, and continuous neurological monitoring is encouraged to quickly identify any complications. As is routine in all institutions, care should be taken to explain the risks, which include death, ischemic or hemorrhagic stroke, access site bleeding requiring transfusion, paralysis, or potential worsening of symptoms weighed against resolution of symptoms by intervention. Low-dose weight-adjusted heparin to maintain an activated clotting time greater than 200 seconds is the procedural anticoagulant of choice for vertebral artery intervention. Bivalirudin is an acceptable alternative in patients with heparin-induced thrombocytopenia.

Step 1. Procedural Planning with Diagnostic Angiography

Using ultrasound guidance, access the femoral artery with a micropuncture needle and 0.018 wire employing the Seldinger technique [7]. Connect the manifold to the micropuncture 4 Fr sheath and perform a femoral angiogram to ensure proper access without complication (optional) or, alternatively, upsize to a 6 Fr femoral sheath over a diagnostic J-wire or Hi-Torque Supra Core guidewire (Abbott vascular, Santa Clara, CA, USA) and perform a femoral angiogram. Insert a 5 Fr or 6 Fr pigtail catheter via a diagnostic J-wire or exchange-length J-wire to perform an aortic arch angiogram in the LAO view (Figure 3.1). The pigtail should be placed in the ascending aorta just proximal to the innominate artery. This view is performed to rule out anomalous vertebral artery origin. Using a 0.035 glidewire or J-wire, insert a 5 Fr Berenstein catheter via the femoral access sheath (alternatively, a 5 Fr or 6 Fr Judkins right, internal mammary, or Vitek curve catheters are acceptable). If brachial or radial access is obtained, a multipurpose or Judkins right catheter is used instead. Carefully engage the vertebral artery ostium, while monitoring continuous pressure. Perform high-quality angiograms of all four supra-aortic main vessels, laying out vertebral artery anatomy (Figure 3.2), especially the target lesion (Figure 3.3). Proceed to image the cervical carotid and vertebral arteries and intracranial arteries (Figure 3.4). Digital subtraction techniques are essential when imaging intracranial anatomy. A minimum image intensifier size of 12 in. is necessary to adequately image the intracranial vessels. A complete angiographic evaluation includes an aortic arch and four-vessel study with selective angiography of bilateral carotid and vertebral arteries including intracranial imaging to ensure collateral blood supply and define the circle of Willis. Nonionic, iso-osmolar contrast is used for intracranial angiography. Importantly, femoral access is used 80% of the time. Ipsilateral brachial or radial artery access is used

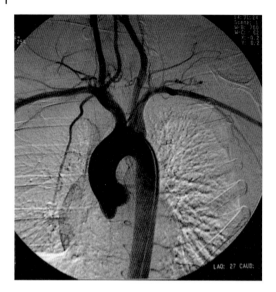

Figure 3.1   Aortic arch angiography showing main supra-aortic vessels.

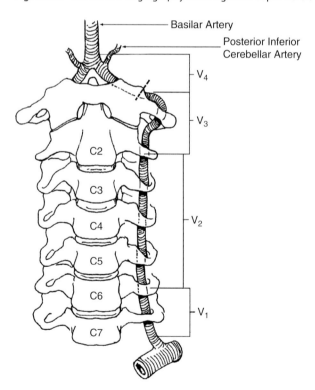

Figure 3.2   Vertebral artery anatomy. *Source:* From Jenkins and Collins (2011).

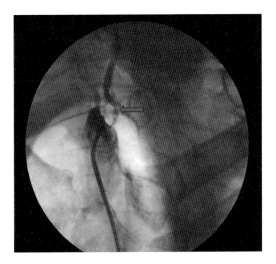

Figure 3.3 Ostial right vertebral artery stenosis (Arrow).

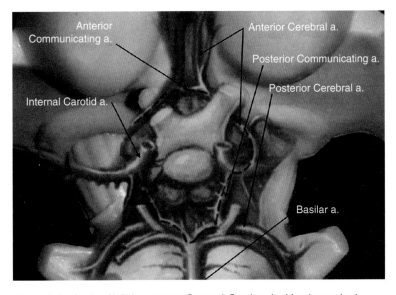

Figure 3.4 Circle of Willis anatomy. *Source:* J. Stephen Jenkins (co-author).

20% of the time if the proximal vertebral artery is acutely angulated when imaged from the femoral access. A combination of femoral and upper extremity access is used in complex cases involving subclavian artery atherosclerotic disease.

A 4 Fr diagnostic catheters do not provide adequate visualization when performing selective vertebral or carotid artery angiography; hence, larger catheters and sheaths should be used.

Step 2. Vertebral Artery Intervention (Percutaneous Transluminal Angioplasty)

Using the usual coronary intervention equipment (wire introducer and hemostasis valve), insert an appropriately sized coronary Rapid exchange (RX) or monorail balloon over a 0.014 soft guidewire. Balloon length is determined by the lesion length and should cover the lesion completely. Balloon diameter should be 0.5 mm less than the reference vessel.

The reference vessel diameter should be determined with quantitative angiography. After correct positioning is confirmed with a contrast test under fluoroscopy, dilate the lesion completely by inflating the balloon (following the balloon rated burst pressure recommendation to avoid complication) (Figure 3.5). Remove the balloon and with the guidewire still distal to the lesion, perform an angiogram of the dilated lesion to assess for successful and satisfactory lesion dilatation (Figure 3.6). Importantly, a 6–8 Fr Judkins right or multipurpose guiding catheter can be used to perform most vertebral interventions. If intervention will be performed, the operator may upsize the 6 Fr sheath for an 8 Fr sheath over a Supra Core wire, Wholey wire 0.035-in. exchange-length wire (Mallinckrodt, St. Louis, MO, USA) or diagnostic J-wire. Balloon length is determined by the lesion length and should cover the lesion completely. Balloon diameter should be 0.5 mm less than the reference vessel. An EPD should be used in all vertebral arteries with an adequate landing zone distal to the index lesion. This is off-label, as there is no embolic protection device with US Food and Drug Administration (FDA) approval

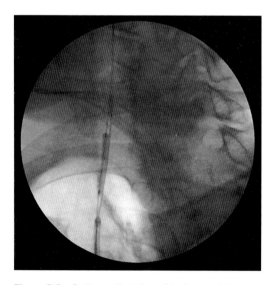

Figure 3.5 Balloon dilatation of lesion: multipurpose guide and 0.014 guidewire with 3.5 × 20 angioplasty balloon.

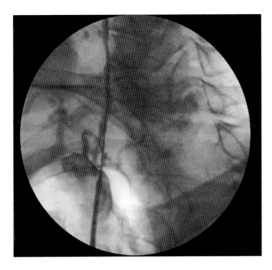

Figure 3.6   Result of balloon angioplasty – Not satisfactory result.

for use in the vertebral artery. In our previously published retrospective series (Jenkins JACC 2010 we did not use embolic protection devices), there were 0% stroke and 1% TIA.

Step 3. Vertebral Artery Intervention (Stenting)

If after balloon dilatation of the lesion, there is suboptimal result, dissection, or perforation the operator should proceed to stenting: Over a 0.014 guidewire, insert a balloon expandable coronary or peripheral stent over the lesion. Extend the stent flush with 1–2 mm into the subclavian artery if stenting the proximal vertebral artery to assure complete coverage of the ostium. A Flash Balloon (Cordis, Santa Clara, CA, USA) may be useful to prevent future procedures in the subclavian artery from damaging the vertebral stent. Ensure the stent is well seated with fluoroscopy prior to deployment (Figure 3.7). Both balloon expandable and self-expanding stents are acceptable in the V1 and V2 segments if the vertebral artery ostium is not involved. Balloon expandable coronary or peripheral stents on a 0.014 platform work well in the VO position. One needs to be certain that the proximal portion of the stent covers the vertebral ostium. It is not uncommon for the proximal stent to extend into the subclavian artery by 1–2 mm. If extension into the subclavian artery is excessive, a Flash Balloon may be used to flair the ostium. Inflate and deploy the stent appropriately (Figure 3.8). The guidewire should always be kept within view during the procedure to prevent perforation and causing fatal intracranial hemorrhage. Care should be exercised when using

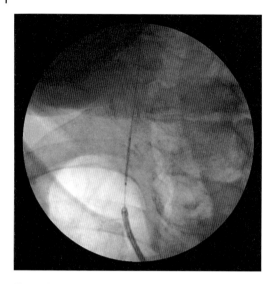

Figure 3.7 4.0 × 23 mm Stent positioned 2 mm proximal to vertebral artery ostium.

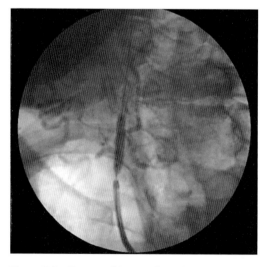

Figure 3.8 Stent position confirmation during deployment.

a hydrophilic guidewire. Depending on the size of stents, deploy with 6–8 atm inflations. If high-pressure post-dilation will be carried out, withdraw the balloon slightly to prevent distal edge dissection. After stent deployment, angiography should be performed to include the posterior intracranial circulation and exclude distal dissection or vessel perforation (Figure 3.9).

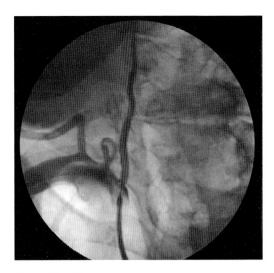

Figure 3.9   Final result.

Table 3.1   Major adverse events associated with vertebral angioplasty.

Event	Frequency (%)
TIA	1–2%
Major stroke	1–2%
MI	0%
Death	<1%

Source: Data from Eberhardt et al. (2006); Jenkins et al. (2010).

Importantly, extend the stent into the subclavian artery by 1–2 mm if stenting the proximal vertebral artery to assure complete coverage of the ostium. Ensure with fluoroscopy that the stent is well seated prior to deployment. The guidewire should always be kept within view during the procedure to prevent perforation and causing fatal intracranial hemorrhage. Care should be exercised when using a hydrophilic guidewire. Multiple catheters, guidewires, balloons, and stents can be used in vertebral interventions not limited to those described in this guide (Table 3.1).

Management of Potential Complications

A team approach including a neurologist, neurointerventional radiologist, and a cardiologist is recommended to assist the interventionalist in dealing with any complications that may arise. Periprocedural complications of vertebral artery

Table 3.2 Interventional tools.

	Size	Device
Guide catheter	6-Fr	Envoy
		Judkins right
		Internal mammary
		Multipurpose
Guidewires	0.014 in.	Balance middle weight (Abbott)
		Wisper (Abbott)
		Choice PT (Cordis)
Embolic protection	4–6 mm	Filterwire (BSC)
Stents balloon expandable	3–6 mm	Vision (Abbott)
		RX Herculink Elite (Abbott)
		Express renal/biliary SD (BSC)
		Multi-link ultra coronary stent (Cordis)
Stents self-expanding	4–7 mm	Xpert pro peripheral stent (Abbott)

Source: Jenkins Vertebral artery interventions, Adapted from Schillinger and Minar (2010) [6].

stenting include both adverse events associated with vertebral angioplasty as well as all other complications that accompany percutaneous procedures. Management of these complications requires repeat imaging to treat mechanical complications of the angioplasty procedure or catheter-directed thrombolysis for thromboembolic events. The frequencies of these major adverse events are quite low (Table 3.2) [5, 8].

Postprocedural Care

1) Plavix (75 mg daily) should be continued for one month after the procedure if bare-metal stents are used with aspirin (81 mg daily) to be continued indefinitely. If drug-eluting stents are used, dual antiplatelet therapy should be continued six months to one year.
2) Dual antiplatelet therapy is frequently continued indefinitely with the use of drug-eluting stents to prevent the occurrence of late stent thrombosis.
3) Duplex ultrasound should be performed at 3, 6, and 12 months and yearly thereafter, if VBI symptoms resolve. Patients with recurrent symptoms should undergo repeat angiography to identify restenosis or progression of atherosclerotic disease.

References

1 Markus, H.S., Larsson, S.C., Kuker, S.C. et al. (2018). Stenting for symptomatic vertebral artery stenosis: the vertebral artery ischaemia stenting trial. *J. Vasc. Surg.* 67 (3): 986.

2 Markus, H.S., Larsson, S.C., Kuker, W. et al. (2017 Sep 19). Stenting for symptomatic vertebral artery stenosis. *Neurology* 89 (12): 1229.

3 (2001). Endovascular versus surgical treatment in patients with carotid stenosis in the carotid and vertebral artery transluminal angioplasty study (CAVATAS): a randomised trial. *The Lancet* 357 (9270): 1729–1737.

4 Jenkins, J.S. (2014). Percutaneous treatment of vertebral artery stenosis. *Interv. Cardiol. Clin.* 3 (1): 115–122.

5 Jenkins, J.S., Patel, S.N., White, C.J. et al. (2010). Endovascular stenting for vertebral artery stenosis. *J. Am. Coll. Cardiol.* 55 (6): 538–542.

6 Schillinger, M. and Minar, E. (2010). *Complex Cases in Peripheral Vascular Interventions*, 308. CRC Press.

7 Garry, B.P. and Bivens, H.E. (1988). The Seldinger technique. *J. Cardiothorac. Anesth.* 2 (3): 403.

8 Eberhardt, O., Naegele, T., Raygrotzki, S. et al. (2006). Stenting of vertebrobasilar arteries in symptomatic atherosclerotic disease and acute occlusion: case series and review of the literature. *J. Vasc. Surg.* 43 (6): 1145–1154.

4

Endovascular Repair of Thoracic Aortic Aneurysms

Catheter-Based Therapy

John Denesopolis, Patricia Yau, and Aksim G. Rivera

Department of Surgery (Vascular Surgery), Albert Einstein College of Medicine-Jacobi Medical Center, Bronx, NY, USA

Introduction

Thoracic aortic pathology has increasingly become a major cause of mortality in the United States, accounting for at least 13 000 deaths annually, with incidence 5.6–10.4 cases per 100 000 people. Thoracic aortic aneurysm (TAA) is predominantly a disease of the older people, with risk factors similar to that of patients with abdominal aortic aneurysm (AAA), i.e. smoking, hypertension, and atherosclerotic disease. The majority are degenerative in etiology, though approximately 20% are sequelae of chronic aortic dissection. Most diagnosed thoracic aortic and thoracoabdominal aortic aneurysms (TAAA) are not symptomatic, and are incidentally noted on imaging obtained for unrelated reasons [1].

The use of endovascular stent grafting, first popularized for AAAs, has now become a mainstay of treatment for TAA. Thoracic endovascular aortic repair (TEVAR) has been shown to have clear benefit in morbidity and mortality to open repair in more recent literature. In patients with less-than-ideal anatomy, e.g. involvement of major aortic branches, tortuous anatomy, large diameter neck, etc., the advantage of endovascular repair over open repair becomes less pronounced. However, with more sophisticated technology, as well as the advent of fenestrated, branching, and hybrid techniques, the use of TEVAR in

Endovascular Interventions: A Step-by-Step Approach, First Edition. Edited by Jose M. Wiley, Cristina Sanina, George D. Dangas, and Prakash Krishnan.
© 2023 John Wiley & Sons Ltd. Published 2023 by John Wiley & Sons Ltd.

patients with complex aortic pathology has proven to be safe, effective, and durable. Additionally, the indications for use of TEVAR have expanded to include blunt traumatic aortic injury, aortic dissection, and acute aortic syndromes.

Relevant Anatomy

Aortic Anatomy

The thoracic aorta consists of four main parts: the aortic root, the ascending thoracic aorta, the aortic arch, and the descending thoracic aorta. The aorta normally enlarges as it progresses distally, and moves posterolaterally in the proximal portion, and anteromedially closer to the diaphragm. Aneurysmal dilatation is defined as $1.5 \times$ normal diameter; normal diameter for the descending aorta is 2.0–2.3 cm. Aneurysm morphology is characterized as fusiform or saccular, with saccular aneurysms having a higher risk of rupture.

Crawford Classification for TAA/TAAA

Type I: arises from above 6th intercostal space, extends to above the renal arteries
Type II: arises above 6th intercostal space, extends distal to the renal arteries
Type III: arises in the distal half of the descending thoracic aorta (below the 6th intercostal space), extends into the abdominal aorta
Type IV: limited to abdominal aorta (diaphragm to aortic bifurcation)
Type V: distal half of descending thoracic aorta to visceral abdominal aorta

Landing Zones (Figure 4.1)

Zone 0: proximal to innominate artery
Zone 1: proximal to CCA
Zone 2: proximal to origin of left SCA
Zone 3: proximal descending aorta (<2 cm from left SCA)
Zone 4: 2 cm distal to SCA, to proximal half of descending thoracic aorta (T6)
Zone 5: distal half descending thoracic aorta to celiac artery
Zone 6: celiac to SMA
Zone 7: SMA to suprarenal aorta
Zone 8: perirenal aorta
Zone 9: infrarenal aorta
Zone 10: common iliac arteries
Zone 11: external iliac arteries

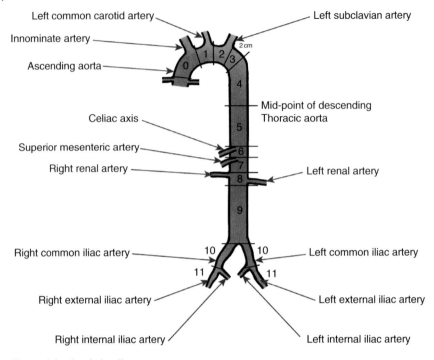

Figure 4.1 Aortic landing ones.

Preoperative planning for TEVAR requires consideration of proximal and distal landing zones and the potential for coverage of major aortic branches. At least 20 mm of proximal and distal landing zone is recommended to allow adequate seal. If there is significant tortuosity, a longer sealing zone may be desired.

Consideration of aortoiliac anatomy is important for determining arterial access and potential need for iliac conduit for graft delivery. The right iliac artery is the preferred route of graft delivery. The access vessel should be at least 7 mm in diameter. If there is not an adequately sized vessel, or if there is significant athero-sclerotic disease, an iliac conduit may be required for device delivery. In rare cases where the entire iliac system is diseased, direct aortic access or an iliac endoconduit may be used (described below).

Implication of Aortic Anatomy on Spinal Perfusion

Spinal cord ischemia is a particularly devastating complication that may occur in 3–7% of patients following TEVAR. Rates of spinal cord ischemia have remained the same despite increasing use of endovascular repair. The blood supply to the spinal cord consists of the posterior spinal arteries (arising from the vertebral or posterior inferior cerebellar arteries), anterior spinal artery (originates from the vertebral arteries), and supported by the artery of Adamkiewicz (usually takes off between T8 and L2). This network is reinforced by collaterals from the radicular arteries, which are supplied by inflow vessels: subclavian/vertebrals, thyrocervical and costocervical trunks, intercostals, lumbar arteries, and branches of hypogastric. Thus, the risk of spinal cord ischemia is increased with coverage of the left SCA and coverage of the hypogastric. Increased length of aortic coverage, renal insufficiency, prior abdominal aortic repair, and intraoperative hypotension are other risk factors for spinal cord ischemia. Coverage of the left SCA also significantly increases the risk of stroke, particularly in 60% of patients with a dominant left vertebral artery. Revascularization of the left SCA, usually by carotid to subclavian bypass, is mandatory in these patients if the left SCA is covered. If surgical reconstruction is contraindicated and left SCA coverage is anticipated, preoperative evaluation should include imaging to assess patency of the right vertebral artery and continuity of the circle of Willis.

Indications/Contraindications to Procedure

Indications

Asymptomatic TAA/TAAA
The goal of surgical intervention for asymptomatic TAA/TAAA is the prevention of rupture. The most important risk factors for rupture for TAAs are size, rate of expansion, and saccular morphology. Current criteria for elective repair of asymptomatic TAA are maximum diameter >5.5 or growth >5 mm over six months [2].

Blunt Aortic Injury (BAI)
TEVAR has largely replaced open repair as first-line surgical management for BAI. Traditionally, the goal has been for definitive surgical repair as early as possible; however, recent data has shown decreased risk of mortality in delayed (>24 hours) repair.

Acute Aortic Syndromes
Type B aortic dissection (TBAD): First-line treatment for uncomplicated TBAD continues to be medical management with tight blood pressure control. However, TBAD with malperfusion may be treated with TEVAR with the goal of sealing the proximal tear and allowing reexpansion of the true lumen [3, 4]. Between 40 and 60% of TBAD which are treated with medical management undergo aneurysmal degeneration of the false lumen, requiring surgical intervention. There may be a

role for elective TEVAR in the subacute period. The INSTEAD trial investigated treatment of subacute TBAD, comparing those treated with endograft and medical management. The data revealed that there was no difference in all cause mortality or aortic-related mortality between the two groups, and the risk of the combined secondary outcome of rupture and progression of disease was the same.

Penetrating aortic ulcer (PAU) and Intramural hemorrhage (IMH): PAU and intramural hematoma are two entities that are separate from TBAD but may present with similar symptoms of acute chest/back pain associated with hypertension. Some believe that the three entities are on the same spectrum of disease; however, the natural progression between the three pathologies is unknown. A PAU, as the name implies, is an atherosclerotic ulcer on the aortic wall that erodes into the aortic wall, whereas an intramural hematoma is a collection of blood between the intima and the media. The natural history of these pathologies is not as well understood as dissection, and thus the indications for and timing of surgical intervention are still under investigation.

Contraindications/Caveats

In patients with ideal anatomy, TEVAR seems to be the preferred option for most cases, with current literature demonstrating reduced morbidity and mortality. However, data regarding long-term (lifelong) follow-up for TEVAR patients is scarce. In younger, healthier patients with a longer life expectancy, consideration can be made for open repair. As stated previously, the presence of challenging anatomy, such as involvement of major aortic branches, large diameter neck, significant angulation, or circumferential thrombus within the seal zones, may make endovascular repair more difficult. In these cases, a careful risk–benefit assessment must be made, taking into account patient comorbidities and surgeon experience. Endovascular stent grafting for infected TAA is not recommended, but can be considered for patients who are poor surgical candidates.

Available Endografts

1) Cook Zenith Alpha (Figure 4.2):
   A) Stent/graft material:
      – Nitinol
      – Tightly woven Dacron
   B) Lengths (cm):
      – Proximal straight: 10.5–23.3
      – Proximal with 4 mm taper: 10.8–23.3
      – Distal: 14.2–21.1
      – Distal extension: 9.1–11.2

C) Diameter (mm):
  - Straight proximal: 24–46
  - Proximal with 4 mm taper: 30–46
  - Distal: 28–46
D) Delivery sheath (Inner diameter):
  - 16, 18, 20 Fr
E) Instructions for use:
  - Isolated lesions of the descending thoracic aorta having vascular anatomy suitable for endovascular repair:
    • Iliac/femoral anatomy that is suitable for access with the required introduction systems
    • Nonaneurysmal aortic segments (fixation sites) proximal and distal to the thoracic lesion
    • Length of at least 20 mm
    • Diameter measured outer wall to outer wall of no greater than 42 mm and no less than 15 mm.

2) Cook TX2 Dissection Graft (Figure 4.3):
  A) Stent/graft material:
    - Stainless steel
    - Standard Dacron
  B) Lengths (cm):
    - Straight proximal: 7.9–21.8
    - Proximal with 4 mm taper: 15.4–21
    - Proximal with 8 mm taper: 15.6–21
  C) Diameter (mm):
    - Proximal straight: 22–42

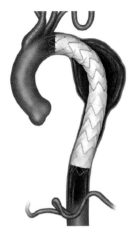

Figure 4.2 Cook Zenith Alpha Graft.

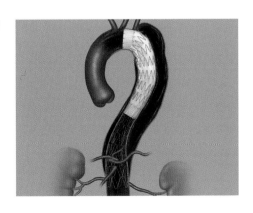

Figure 4.3 Cook TX2 graft and dissection stent.

- Proximal with 4 mm taper: 32–42
- Proximal with 8 mm taper: 32–42

D) Delivery sheath (Inner diameter*):
  - 20–22 Fr

E) Instructions for use:
  - Treatment of patients with atherosclerotic aneurysms, symptomatic acute or chronic dissections, contained ruptures, growing aneurysms, and/or resulting in distal ischemia, in the descending thoracic aorta having vascular morphology suitable for endovascular repair:
    - Adequate iliac/femoral access compatible with the required introduction systems
    - Radius of curvature greater than 35 mm along the entire length of aorta intended to be treated
    - Nonaneurysmal aortic segments (fixation sites) proximal and distal to the aneurysm:
      o With a length of at least 20 mm
      o With a diameter measured outer wall to outer wall of no greater than 38 mm and no less than 20 mm
      o With an angle less than 45°.

3) Cook TX2 Dissection Stent:
   A) Stent material
     - Nitinol
   B) Lengths (cm):
     - 8, 12, 18, 18.5
   C) Diameters (mm):
     - 36, 46
   D) Delivery sheath (Inner diameter*)
     - 16 Fr
   E) Instructions for use:
     - Intended to be used as a distal component to provide support to delaminated segments of nonaneurysmal aorta with dissection distal to a Zenith TX2 Dissection Endovascular Graft in the descending thoracic aorta having vascular morphology suitable for endovascular repair:
       - Aortic fixation site diameter 20–38 mm (measured outer wall to outer wall)
       - Radius of curvature >35 mm along the length of aorta that is intended to be treated
       - Localized angulation <45°.

4) Gore cTAG with Active Control (Figure 4.4):
   A) Stent/graft material:
     - Nitinol
     - ePTFE

(a)

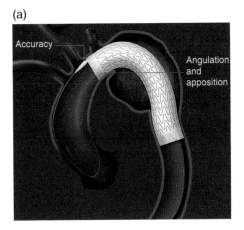

(b)

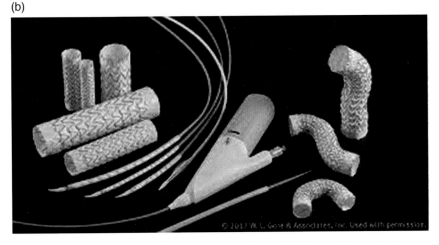

Figure 4.4 (a) and (b) Gore cTAG endoprosthesis. *Source:* W. L. Gore & Associates, Inc.

B) Lengths (cm):
 – 10, 15, 20
C) Diameter (mm):
 – Straight: 21, 26, 28, 31, 34, 37, 40, 45
 – Tapered: 26×21, 31×26
D) Delivery sheath (Inner diameter):
 – 18, 20, 22, 24 Fr
E) Instructions for use:
 Repair of aneurysms of the descending thoracic aorta in patients who have appropriate anatomy:

- Adequate iliac/femoral access
- Aortic inner diameter in the range of 23–37 mm
- 2 cm nonaneurysmal aorta proximal and distal to the aneurysm.

5) Terumo Aortic Relay (Figure 4.5):
  A) Stent/graft material:
    – Nitinol
    – PTFE sutures, woven polyester graft
  B) Lengths (cm):
    – Straight: 10, 15, 20, 25
    – 4 mm Tapered: 15, 20, 25
  C) Diameter (mm):
    – Straight: 22–46
    – Proximal with 4 mm taper: 28–46
  D) Delivery sheath (Outer diameter):
    – 22, 23, 24, 25, 26 Fr
  E) Instructions for use:
    Repair of fusiform aneurysms and saccular aneurysms/penetrating athero-sclerotic ulcers in the descending thoracic aorta in patients having appropriate anatomy:

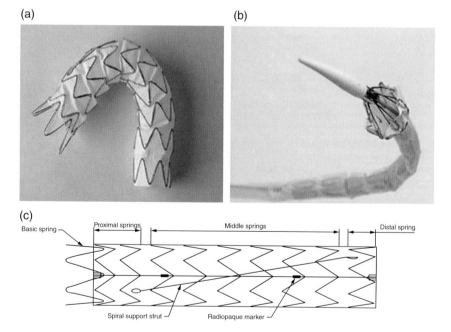

Figure 4.5 Terumo relay aortic graft. *Source:* Elsevier Inc.

- Iliac or femoral access vessel morphology that is compatible with vascular access techniques, devices, and/or accessories
- Nonaneurysmal aortic neck diameter in the range of 19–42 mm
- Nonaneurysmal proximal aortic neck length between 15 and 25 mm
- Nonaneurysmal distal aortic neck length between 25 and 30 mm.

6) Medtronic Valiant (Figure 4.6):
   A) Stent/graft material:
      – Nitinol
      – Woven polyester
   B) Length (cm):
      – Straight: 5.5, 6, 10, 17.5, 22.5
      – Tapered: 17.5, 18.5, 20
   C) Diameter (mm):
      – Straight: 20, 22, 25, 28, 31, 34, 37, 40, 43, 46
      – Tapered: 25, 28, 31, 34, 37, 40, 43, 46
   D) Delivery sheath (Outer diameter):
      – 18, 20, 22 Fr
   E) Instructions for use:
      Repair of all lesions of the descending thoracic aorta in patients having the appropriate anatomy:
      - Iliac or femoral artery access vessel morphology that is compatible with vascular access techniques, devices, or accessories

Figure 4.6 Medtronic valiant thoracic endograft. *Source:* Vascular News.

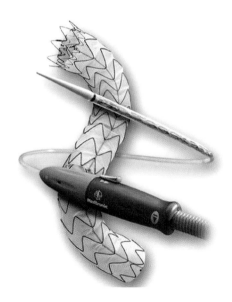

- Nonaneurysmal aortic diameter in the range of 18–42 mm (fusiform and saccular aneurysms/penetrating ulcers), or 18–44 mm (blunt traumatic aortic injuries), or 20–44 mm (dissections)
- Nonaneurysmal aorta proximal and distal neck lengths ≥20 mm (fusiform and saccular aneurysms/penetrating ulcers), landing zone ≥20 mm proximal to the primary entry tear (blunt traumatic aortic injuries, dissections)
- The proximal extent of the landing zone must not be dissected.

Preoperative Evaluation

The evaluation of the patient with TAA should begin with a thorough history and physical examination. In particular, history of cardiac, pulmonary, and renal disease should be elicited. Routine preoperative laboratory testing, EKG, and chest radiography should be performed.

Cardiac evaluation: Due to the advanced age of the population and prevalence of atherosclerotic risk factors, a significant number of patients with TAA/TAAA have concomitant cardiac disease. Preoperative echocardiogram can be useful for assessing myocardial and valvular function; however, the benefit of routine use of cardiac echo in all TEVAR patients is controversial. Patients who have signs or symptoms of cardiac disease should undergo further evaluation to determine the presence and extent of coronary artery disease. If indicated, patients should undergo coronary revascularization prior to or during TEVAR.

Pulmonary evaluation: The presence of COPD is directly associated with increased perioperative mortality after TEVAR. Preoperative testing including pulmonary function tests and arterial blood gas should be routinely performed. Smoking cessation, if applicable, should be encouraged. Compliance to prescribed inhalers should be ensured as this has been directly linked to mortality in TEVAR patients.

Renal evaluation: Renal failure is common following TEVAR, and is associated with postoperative nonrenal complications. Additionally, preoperative chronic renal insufficiency is a strong risk factor for postoperative morbidity and mortality. All patients should undergo careful evaluation of renal function, with renal artery duplex ultrasound if warranted. If severe renal artery occlusive disease is present, preoperative or intraoperative revascularization may be considered. Preoperative intravenous hydration should be strongly considered in high-risk patients.

Imaging: CTA including the aortic arch, chest, abdomen, and pelvis should be obtained. Three-dimensional reconstructions help visualize tortuosity of the vessels. Particular attention should be paid to arch anatomy as well as the positioning of the vertebral arteries if there is involvement of zones 0, 1, or 2. If the patient is at higher risk for spinal cord ischemia, assessment of pelvic perfusion is imperative.

Positioning and Intraoperative Monitoring Needs

General anesthesia with endotracheal intubation is recommended; however, it can be done under sedation or with local in cases where general anesthesia may not be tolerated. Cardiac anesthesia team strongly recommended, as they can perform intraoperative ECHO to confirm no proximal extension of dissection.

Arterial line is strongly recommended for intraoperative blood pressure monitoring and as an added caveat, its tracing can estimate the degree of malperfusion of the left arm if the left subclavian needs to be covered. Spinal drain based on extent of coverage and if elective in order to decrease the incidence of spinal cord ischemia as coverage of the subclavian, intercostals, and/or spinal artery may occur based on anatomic needs of the case. Temperature Probe foley to ensure both appropriate urine production intraoperative and post op as well as to monitor intraoperative temperature so as to avoid hypothermia and coagulopathy.

Patient is positioned supine on an angiography table. If using a Stille bed, ensure that the T of the bed is at the patient's feet rather than at the head so as to visualize the entire aorta. In a standard TEVAR case, a standard prep may involve preparing both groins and proximal thighs as well as the abdomen from the umbilicus down in case more proximal or distal control must be obtained.

If access vessels are too small, an iliac conduit may be required:

a) Procedure in which a low abdominal wall incision is created to gain access to the common, internal, and external iliac arteries.
b) Depending on durability of vessels, a graft is anastomosed in an end-to-side or end-to-end configuration.
c) An incision is made on the graft and a long 8 Fr sheath can be introduced and secured with umbilical tape.
d) The remainder of the endograft deployment is the same as a standard TEVAR which is described below.
e) At the end of the case, the graft is dealt with in one of several ways:
  1) Tying off the graft as a stump.
  2) Sewing the distal end of the conduit to more distal segment of iliac as an interposition graft.
  3) Passing the graft under the inguinal ligament and performing end-to-side anastomosis to the common femoral artery (ideal if future cannulation is anticipated).

If subclavian coverage is planned in an elective case and subclavian revascularization is required, the head should be turned toward the right and the neck and clavicular region should be prepped into the field. If thoracoabdominal aneurysm case then depending on the extent of arch disease, the chest, bilateral neck, abdomen, and left arm should be prepped into the field.

Procedural Steps

Deployment of specific grafts varies from product to product. Below is a brief general guide for a standard TEVAR:

Step 1. Ultrasound guided bilateral access initially with 5–7 Fr on the contralateral side and 7 Fr on the working side.

Step 2. Confirm access wire in each femoral artery using fluoroscopy.

Access should be in the top half/top third of the femoral head to make manual pressure easier. Confirmatory shot can be anterior or slightly anterior oblique (Figure 4.7).

Step 3. A guidewire and angled catheter are used to enter the abdominal aorta and under fluoroscopy the wire and catheter are guided into the thoracic aorta. A wire exchange for a stiff wire should be performed at this time with the

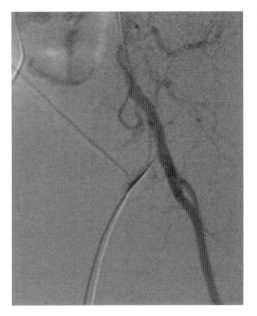

Figure 4.7 Confirmation of common femoral cannulation.

angled catheter in place. As with all catheter, sheath, and wire exchanges described here and in other chapters, it is critical to perform appropriate over wire and through catheter exchanges for all of your equipment so as to keep the equipment in the appropriate position and to avoid further damage to the aortic wall.

Step 4. Confirmation of wire in true lumen with intravascular ultrasound (IVUS) (optional but recommended for dissections) (Figure 4.8).

Step 5. Perclose on operative side if this is done completely percutaneously, usual recommendation is for deployment of two devices at 10 o'clock and 2 o'clock positions.

Step 6. Advancement of marked diagnostic catheter (usually a pigtail or contra catheter depending on supplies at facility) to shoot diagnostic aortogram on contralateral side (Figure 4.9).

This step is critical as this is the last time possible for accurate sizing of the aortic lumen diameter as well as length from the subclavian artery, entry tear, and distal landing zone. IVUS can be used in this step as well to further confirm size and proximal extent of dissection. It is generally recommended to oversize the stent-graft about 5–10%. Ventilation should be held during any diagnostic shots for appropriate sizing.

Step 7. Exchange introducer sheath for device sheath on working side.

Step 8. Advance over wire into thoracic aorta and confirm placement prior to deployment.

Step 9. Deploy graft:

Figure 4.8 Intravascular ultrasound displaying true and false lumen (probe in compressed true lumen).

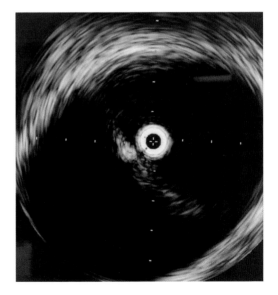

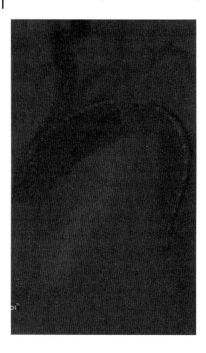

Figure 4.9 Arch aortogram to identify seal zone.

If intubated and mechanically ventilated, the respirations should be held for accurate placement. Systolic blood pressure during this step should be maintained at 100 mmHg so as to avoid graft motion during deployment. All of the endografts listed above are self-expanding, and balloon molding is neither needed nor is it generally recommended as this may further damage an already vulnerable aortic wall.

Step 10. Completion shots (Figure 4.10):

After deployment, this is the most important step as adequacy of repair and prevention of further aortic degeneration requires correction of endoleaks. This step is also critical to ensure that the graft did not move during placement and that there is appropriate filling of the subclavian (assuming it was not intentionally covered), distal thoracic aorta, and the abdominal aorta and run-off. If dissection extends into visceral aorta, consider using dissection stent to promote aortic modeling.

Step 11. If any type 1 or type 3 endoleaks are present, extend proximally and distally or provide more overlap as seen fit to correct them or use a large diameter balloon to better seal the graft to the aortic wall proximally or distally (Figure 4.11).

Step 12. Remove device and deploy the previously placed perclose devices on the large sheath side.

(a)

(b)

(c)

(d)

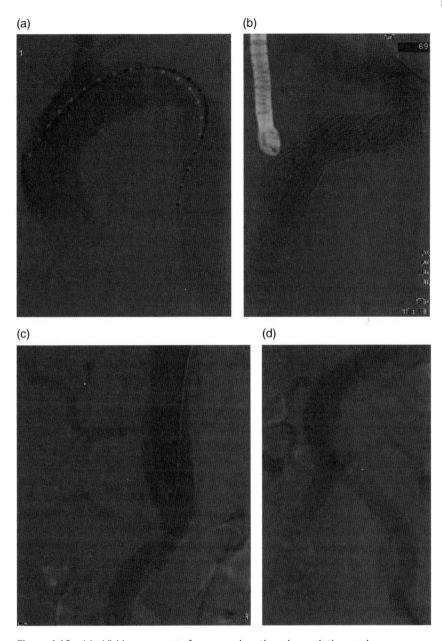

Figure 4.10   (a)–(d) Measurement of coverage length and completion angiogram.

(a)   (b)   (c)

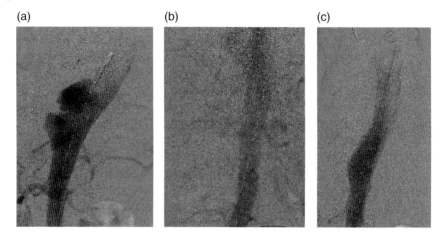

Figure 4.11 (a)–(c) Treatment of penetrating aortic ulcer, initial endoleak, and complete resolution with distal balloon insufflation.

Step 13. Manual pressure or percutaneous closure device on the contralateral side.If manual pressure is applied, then a general rule of thumb is to hold 5 minutes of pressure for each Fr size (i.e. 6 Fr sheath gets 30 minutes of pressure).

Step 14. Check distal pulses to confirm no distal embolization.

Postoperative Course/Surveillance

Monitored Setting

In elective surgery admit TEVAR cases that do not require spinal drain or IV drip, anti-impulse control a surgical step down unit or telemetry unit may be sufficient. In acute settings such as trauma, rupture, or acute dissection, postoperative monitoring should occur in an ICU setting as these patients will likely have comorbid injuries, an arterial line, a spinal drain, and/or require IV drip blood pressure medications.

Spinal Drain

For any nonemergent cases requiring coverage of >20 cm of aortic length, anticipated coverage of T8 or lower, coverage of the subclavian, or prior abdominal aortic stent-graft placement, a spinal drain is recommended to decrease the incidence of spinal cord ischemia and its neurologic sequelae. In order to drive the hydrostatic pressure to be high enough for adequate spinal cord perfusion, two criteria are to be met: (i) systolic blood pressure >100 mmHg (without approaching hypertension that could further damage the aortic wall) and (ii) intrathecal pressure <10 mmHg.

Generally speaking, a spinal drain is kept clamped at 10 mmHg and every hour 10 cc or so of fluid is allowed to drain. If the patient develops headaches or lower extremity symptoms, the drain is opened and allowed to drain until symptoms resolve. Spinal drains should be removed within 24–72 hours of placement. It is important to note that, if the patient was on anticoagulation for any reason, it should be held for the appropriate half-life clearance so as to avoid any bleeding complications.

Blood Pressure Control

As stated above when discussing spinal drains, blood pressure control is paramount in the perioperative period as well as in the patient's eventual lifelong postoperative course. In the preoperative course, blood pressure goals for patients with dissection disease are generally recommended to be in the normotensive range. If the patient does not have signs of malperfusion and symptoms are absent with adequate blood pressure management, it may be acceptable to follow these patients clinically without placement of stent-graft. Symptomatic dissections despite adequate blood pressure control or dissections with signs of malperfusion (mesenteric ischemia, renal ischemia, ischemic hepatopathy, or lower extremity ischemia) require immediate treatment. In patients with ruptured thoracic aorta, blood pressure resuscitative goals are to make sure that the patient is adequately perfusing the brain and vital organs in anticipation of emergent surgical repair. Blood pressure goals for patients with traumatic aortic injury are similar to those of spontaneous dissection, excluding patients with transected aortas.

Arm Ischemia Symptoms

Arm ischemia is a rare but preventable/treatable sequelae that can arise in about 18% of patients undergoing subclavian coverage without preoperative revasculation [5]. It is highly recommended for elective cases where it is known that the patient will require coverage of the subclavian that a carotid subclavian bypass or a carotid subclavian transposition be performed prior to stent-graft placement. Decision of carotid subclavian bypass versus transposition is highly based on prior coronary artery bypass. Using a LIMA conduit as a transposition will compromise flow to the LIMA bypass during the procedure and can cause a myocardial infarction.

The Society for Vascular Surgery (SVS) has laid out specific guidelines with regard to coverage of the subclavian artery which are easily accessible on the SVS guidelines smartphone application. In emergent cases, the subclavian should be covered if needed so as to avoid type 1a endoleaks and careful postoperative monitoring of arm ischemia symptoms must occur. If the patient develops significant ischemic symptoms of the hand after coverage of the subclavian, revascularization should be performed. In patients who need elective TEVAR where coverage of the subclavian will be needed for appropriate seal, a preoperative subclavian revascularization is suggested.

CTA Surveillance/Endoleak Types

There is no general consensus for exact timing of CTA in the postoperative period or long-term surveillance. Therefore, it is up to physicians to have their own standard for timing of CTA. Many providers obtain CT scans at 1 month, 2 months, 6 months, 12 months, and yearly thereafter to look for aneurysmal degeneration and/or endoleak formation [6]. Some providers obtain CTA prior to discharge in higher risk patients especially in those who presented with acute dissection, trauma, or rupture. Endoleak formation can be a very detrimental factor in the perioperative period and during postoperative surveillance.

There are five distinct endoleak types (Figure 4.12):

1) Type 1: leakage between the graft and aortic wall either at the proximal seal zone (1a) or the distal seal zone (1b)
2) Type 2: back-bleeding from another vessel (subclavian, intercostals)
3) Type 3: inadequate overlap between two stents

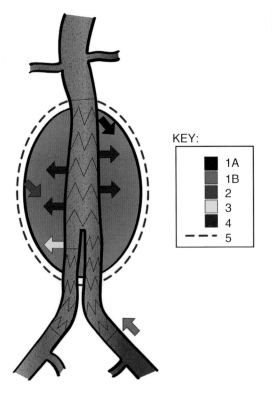

Figure 4.12 Endoleak classification.

KEY:

■	1A
▨	1B
▤	2
□	3
■	4
- - -	5

4) Type 4: increased porosity of the stent-graft
5) Type 5: endotension; increased size of aneurysm sac without other known source.

Types 1 and 3 when seen in the operating room should be repaired as they are technical failures. Type 2 endoleaks if small may be watched as they may revert on their own.

References

1 Faiza, Z. and Sharman, T. (2022). *Thoracic Aorta Aneurysm*. Treasure Island (FL): StatPearls Publishing.
2 Hiratzka, L.F., Bakris, G.L., Beckman, J.A. et al. (2010). 2010 ACCF/AHA/AATS/ ACR/ASA/SCA/SCAI/SIR/STS/SVM guidelines for the diagnosis and management of patients with Thoracic Aortic Disease: A report of the American College of Cardiology. *Circulation* 121 (13): e266–e369.
3 Cambria, R.P., Brewster, D.C., Gertler, J. et al. (1988). Vascular complications associated with spontaneous aortic dissection. *J. Vasc. Surg.* 7 (2): 199–209.
4 Cambria, R.P., Conrad, M.F., Matsumoto, A.H. et al. (2015). Multicenter clinical trial of the conformable stent graft for the treatment of acute, complicated type B dissection. *J. Vasc. Surg.* 62 (2): 271–278.
5 Woo, E.Y., Carpenter, J.P., and Jackson, B.M. (2008). Left subclavian artery coverage during thoracic endovascular aortic repair: A single-center experience. *J. Vasc. Surg.* 48 (3): 555–560.
6 Upchurch, G.R. Jr., Escobar, G.A., Azizzadeh, A. et al. (2021). Society for Vascular Surgery clinical practice guidelines of thoracic endovascular aortic repair for descending thoracic aortic aneurysms. *J. Vasc. Surg.* 73 (1): 55S–83S.

5

Endovascular Abdominal Aortic Aneurysm Repair (EVAR)

John Futchko, Katie MacCallum, and Aksim G. Rivera

Department of Surgery (Vascular Surgery), Albert Einstein College of Medicine-Jacobi Medical Center, Bronx, NY, USA

Introduction

Since it was first described in 1986 [1], endovascular aneurysm repair (EVAR) has become the preferred treatment option for many patients with abdominal aortic aneurysms (AAAs). Multiple studies have shown lower 30-day mortality rates and fewer perioperative complications as compared to open AAA repair [2–4]. Initial concerns regarding durability largely have been alleviated by stent-graft redesign and follow-up trials examining long-term outcomes [5–7]. While overall complication rates are favorable, reintervention rates remain significantly higher than open repair [8].

EVAR requires extensive preoperative planning including appropriate patient selection, detailed imaging, measurements, and graft selection. There are various intraoperative pitfalls, such as vascular access and endoleaks, which the surgeon must be able to identify and troubleshoot. This chapter will provide an overview of the steps of the procedure as well as management of potential issues that may arise.

Patient Selection

Though EVAR is appropriate for most patients, including those otherwise deemed too high-risk for open repair [9], it is not "one size fits all." Various criteria should be considered, particularly anatomic suitability.

One advantage of EVAR over open repair is that it may be performed under anesthesia suited to the patient's needs. General anesthesia is commonly used;

however, either regional (spinal or epidural) or local anesthetic with sedation may be chosen depending on the individual's comorbidities and type of access to be performed. This gives the anesthesiologist relative flexibility as compared to open repair which mandates general anesthesia.

Potential anatomic challenges include a short or severely angled aortic neck, circumferential thrombus, and iliac artery disease, but none of these alone is an absolute contraindication [10–12], particularly with advancements in graft design. Most surgeons consider the character of the neck to be the most important anatomic factor with length, diameter, angulation, and shape all playing important roles in the seal of the proximal graft. Pitfalls related to poor distal vessel quality will be addressed later in the section on vascular access. Preoperative imaging is essential to identifying these issues.

Preoperative Imaging and Measurements

All patients undergoing EVAR will require preoperative imaging. Computed tomography arteriography (CTA) with three-dimensional (3D) reconstructions is the most common and the most useful for planning. Multiple software packages are available, including open source platforms, which enable the surgeon to create precise measurements accounting for the angulation and rotation of the blood vessels involved through centerline reconstructions (Figure 5.1).

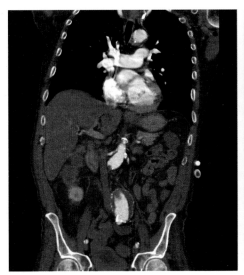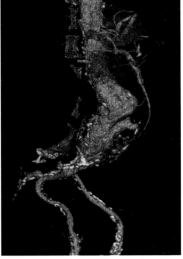

Figure 5.1 Pictured on the left is a traditional CTA coronal view of an infrarenal aneurysm. To the right is 3D reconstruction using available software. Such imaging modalities allow for accurate sizing and pre-operative case planning.

As proper CTA requires intravenous contrast administration, it should be performed judiciously in those patients with chronic kidney disease or concern for contrast allergy. For those who are unable to receive contrast dye, noncontrast CT may be performed. Unfortunately, this will lead to a subpar understanding of the patient's anatomy. Distal occlusive disease or the presence of laminated thrombus may not be appreciated. In these patients, alternative imaging may also be considered such as carbon dioxide angiography [13] or intravascular ultrasound (IVUS). IVUS has also emerged as an essential intraoperative adjunct in performing EVAR for all patients [14].

Graft Selection

Once the surgeon has decided EVAR is a suitable option for an individual patient, the next crucial step is selection of the stent-graft itself. There are multiple companies with devices currently approved for use in the United States and even more in clinical trials. In choosing a graft, one must consider the following key components: profile, graft material, stent material, modularity, ease of use, and range of treatable aortic neck and iliac artery.

The delivery system profile is of particular importance in an aging population or in female patients who may have smaller femoral vessels, thus limiting access. At the time of writing, the smallest delivery sheath system is the Alto™ system (Endologix, Irvine, CA, USA) with an outside diameter (OD) of 15 Fr. All commercially available grafts are currently made with either woven polyester or polytetrafluroethylene (PTFE), similar to materials used during open surgical repair. Proximal fixation may be either infrarenal or suprarenal depending on the inclusion of a bare-metal stent component. Positive fixation may be achieved with additional features such as metal hooks, barbs, anchors, or staples. Additional graft features, such as column support and radial force, will assist with fixation and, ideally, prevent caudal migration over the life of the device.

Manufacturers have selected to produce either bi- or tri-modular devices, with three-piece grafts consisting of the main body and individual iliac limbs as opposed to a main body and iliac piece with a separate contralateral limb piece. Graft selection depends not only on patient anatomy but also on the operator's comfort with the system.

Graft Sizing

Each stent-graft has unique features and thus requires specifically tailored measurements. Most manufacturers have worksheets available to assist in sizing. Generally speaking, grafts should be oversized approximately 10–20% in comparison to the diameter of the aortic neck and iliac arteries to minimize the risk of graft complications, including graft migration and both early and late endoleak during aortic remodeling. While each available endograft device has its own specific instructions for use (IFU), there are several general guidelines in sizing, which can help to determine the complexity of repair required dependent on individual patient anatomy.

Neck Length

One of the most crucial initial measurements in endograft sizing is the distance between the lowest renal artery and the most proximal portion of aneurysmal aorta, typically referred to as the "neck length." This segment of aorta acts as the proximal fixation point for the sealing stents found at the proximal ends of most endograft devices. While there is some variation, as some grafts, such as the Zenith™ (Cook Medical, Bloomington, IN, USA), have bare-metal suprarenal fixation stents, these sealing zone stents provide the necessary wall apposition that leads to aneurysm exclusion. Equally as important is the quality of this aortic segment, as the presence of even mild aneurysmal degeneration or thrombus can lead to intraoperative embolic events, endoleak, or improper aortic remodeling. In general, an aortic neck of at least 15 mm is required for on-label use of most commercially available endografts. However, there are two available devices, the Endurant™ (Medtronic, Minneapolis, MN, USA) graft and Alto graft, which have specific IFU for aneurysms with less than 10 mm of available neck. In the case of the Endurant graft, the use of endoanchors improves apposition and fixation and allows for deployment with as little as 4 mm of available neck length.

Neck Diameter

The measurement of the aortic neck diameter is essential to prevent repair failure and thus equally as important in endograft sizing as neck length. It is typically taken 15 mm from the lowest renal and involves a wall-to-wall measurement in the axial cuts in a plane perpendicular to the course of the aortic lumen; although this may vary based on device. Most device manufacturers recommend oversizing by 10–20% of the aortic diameter. In doing so, current EVAR devices can accommodate aortic diameters between 18 and 32 mm. Oversizing assures adequate wall apposition and reduction of the risk of a type I endoleak. However, overzealous oversizing can result in graft pleating of the fabric and type I endoleak, as well as an increase in late graft migration and aortic neck dilation. This is also important to remember in patients with conical aortic necks. In such cases, most recommend taking the average of both diameters to determine a final endograft stent size.

Branch Vessels

In cases where aneurysmal degeneration extends into the visceral segment and the patient is not suited to open repair, there are several endovascular options falling into three general categories: fenestrated endografts, parallel grafts, and debranching procedures.

Fenestrated endografts have now become commercially available (Zenith). Tailored to an individual patient's anatomy, these custom-made endografts allow for endovascular repair of juxtarenal aneurysms through creation of windows in the endograft designed to align with aortic branch vessels allowing for perfusion (and possible stenting) of visceral arteries. These devices have their own anatomic limitations and offer only limited treatment options in "off-the-shelf" emergent repair situations.

When such devices cannot be utilized, alternative complex endovascular techniques allow for appropriate repair and coverage. Parallel stent-grafts, which include snorkels, periscopes, and chimneys, refer to stent-grafts placed in parallel alongside aortic endografts to allow for perfusion of branch vessels that would otherwise be covered. These repairs are often complicated with endoleak between stent-grafts, so called "gutterleaks," as well as stent-graft thrombosis and type I endoleaks.

Debranching refers to open surgical debranching and bypass of visceral vessels (i.e. celiac, SMA, and renal arteries) to alternative arterial inflow targets (typically iliac arteries) prior to planned endograft coverage.

Aortic Length Measurements

Calculating the aortic length to repair requires several measurements: the lowest renal artery to the aortic bifurcation, the bifurcation to the right hypogastric artery, and the bifurcation to the left hypogastric artery. These measurements can prove challenging, especially in the case of a tortuous aorta or iliac arteries; however, this can be aided with the use of centerline reconstruction software.

For most devices appropriate wall apposition requires at least 10 mm of distance between the aortic bifurcation and the internal iliac artery. The need for longer iliac limbs typically occurs in patients with more tortuous iliacs. Patients with splayed aortic bifurcations may benefit from "balleting" (crossing) the iliac limbs, which also requires longer limb lengths (Figure 5.2).

The distal seal zone along the iliac vessels also plays a critical role in graft sizing. As with proximal fixation, distal fixation typically requires 10–20% oversizing of the measured iliac diameter and is crucial to prevent type IB endoleaks, iliac aneurysmal degeneration, or iliac thrombosis. Iliac arteries less than 7 mm or greater than 25 mm may render endovascular treatment unsuitable. For patients

Figure 5.2 In cases where aortic anatomy is not suitable for on-label device use, graft alteration or "physician-modified endografts" as pictured above can provide an endovascular solution in patients who are otherwise poor candidates for difficult open repairs.

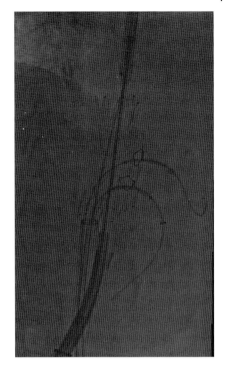

with concurrent iliac occlusive disease, treatment of such lesions should occur prior to endograft placement, as these aortic endografts do not provide the radial force necessary for treatment of stenotic lesions.

For patients with concurrent aneurysmal iliac disease, the Iliac Branch Excluder™ Device (W.L. Gore, Flagstaff, AZ, USA) allows for canalization and preservation of the iliac branch vessels, with exclusion of associated aneurysm. These devices are especially important in patients with occluded contralateral hypogastric vessels.

Step 1. Vascular Access

Percutaneous

Ultrasound-guided percutaneous access has become increasingly routine in both EVAR and thoracic endovascular aortic repair (TEVAR) over the past decade. Multiple peer-reviewed studies have demonstrated that percutaneous access offers patients shorter procedure times and length of stay, as well as decreased postoperative pain and access site wound complications [15, 16]. Percutaneous access can be safely achieved with sheaths up to 24 Fr, which accommodate most commercially available devices. Safe closure of the percutaneous access can be achieved with any of the large-access closure devices available in the market.

As in device sizing and selection, the use of percutaneous access is dependent on patient selection. Those patients with scarred or hostile groins (i.e. previous surgery, radiation, or cancer) tend to benefit from open exposure. Vascular anatomy also plays a key role in decision-making. Patients with a high femoral bifurcation or significant calcific or occlusive iliofemoral disease may not be amenable to percutaneous access. Likewise, patients with small iliofemoral vessels, typically women, usually have limited options for delivery systems. While sometimes overlooked, one ought to remember that vascular access is one of the most crucial portions of the EVAR procedure, the one from which most complications arise. Due to the inherent risks, the ability to convert to open for access and surgical closure must be available.

Initial access is similar to that of a standard lower extremity angiogram and should be performed under ultrasound guidance to limit the risk of complications. The optimal access target is along the anterior surface of the common femoral artery between the inguinal ligament and femoral bifurcation. Arterial cannulation can be obtained using either a standard "single-wall" 18-gauge needle or with a "micropuncture" 21-gauge needle, with wire choice dependent on operator preference and anatomic profile. Access location relative to the femoral head and subsequent placement of guidewire into the iliac system is then confirmed under fluoroscopic imaging.

Open

With the advent and widespread adoption of percutaneous access devices, open access has become less common; however, still has its place in specific patient populations. As mentioned above, open exposure plays an important role to avoid potentially devasting access complications. When performed, a vertical or oblique incision can be utilized. While a vertical incision allows for additional exposure of the femoral vessels, oblique incisions tend to be favored by operators due to decreased rates of wound complications [17].

Iliac Disease and Conduits

Even after successful groin access, iliac occlusive disease may be a major hindrance to endograft deployment. Evaluation of the iliac vessels on preoperative CTA allows for planning sheath navigation and device approach through potentially diseased and tortuous vessels. Wire selection and access during this portion of the procedure is crucial. Any placement of dilator sheaths and larger devices should occur over very stiff wires. Wire selection will be discussed in detail later in the chapter. Additionally, it is crucial to maintain wire placement across the iliac arteries throughout the duration of the case. In many instances, the damage in diseased iliacs occurs with vessel injury or disruption upon removal of a large bore sheath. In these devastating moments, a stiff wire can provide life-saving access.

There are several approaches to iliac occlusive disease, dependent on the degree of disease and device used. Often, focal iliac lesions can be treated prior to sheath insertion with balloon angioplasty. For patients with more significant disease that requires stenting, there are two key concepts to remember. First, these aortic endografts do not provide the radial force to maintain long-term patency in the iliacs, and thus should not be used in lieu of a stent. Second, if stenting is required, it should be done following deployment of the endograft, given the tendency for many bare-metal stents to migrate with repeated manipulation.

There are several endovascular techniques that allow for access in the case of small or diseased iliac arteries. One option is to create an "internal endovascular conduit" by placing oversized, covered stents in the common and external iliac arteries and balloon-expanding them to a sufficient diameter. Another is the use of a recently developed balloon-expandable sheath (SoloPath, Onset Medical Corp, Irvine, CA, USA). The sheath, which contains an incorporated angioplasty balloon, is initially inserted with a size of 14 Fr then expanded to size 24 Fr, enough to accommodate most devices.

In select cases, the use of a surgically placed graft conduit can be performed to completely bypass diseased and calcified iliac and femoral vessels. The conduit should be performed through a right or left oblique retroperitoneal incision. Taking extreme care to stay retroperitoneal, it is possible to expose an adequate segment of common iliac artery to allow for graft anastomosis. An end-to-side anastomosis in the distal common iliac artery with 10 mm prosthetic conduit. The conduit is then tunneled under the inguinal ligament into a femoral counter incision to be used appropriately for the remainder of the procedure. At the completion of the EVAR, the conduit may be either ligated, a small segment left for later access, or anastomosed to the common femoral artery.

Step 2. Imaging

Equipment

Successful access and appropriate device selection mean little without quality fluoroscopy equipment. Many institutions today have at least one "hybrid" room, which combines a contemporary fixed-imaging unit with traditional operating room capabilities. The procedure may also be performed with the traditional "C-arm" fluoroscopy unit. In both situations, the operator must be comfortably using the equipment efficiently and safely.

Neck Angulation

Many infrarenal aneurysmal necks have varying degrees of angulation, often in an anterior orientation. In order to appropriately correct for this and to remove any parallax in the imaging, a degree of adjustment in the fluoroscopy unit is typically required. This can be calculated using the preoperative CTA in a centerline software system and involves creating an angle perpendicular to the neck of the aneurysm.

Renal Arteries

In a similar fashion, the left renal artery typically originates slightly posterior and lateral on the aorta, requiring adjusting the gantry angle with some degree of left anterior oblique (LAO) to allow for adequate imaging. For patients with accessory renal arteries and normal renal function, these can typically be covered with the endograft without the need for embolization.

Step 3. Wires

With bilateral femoral access established, wire access across the diseased aorta must be achieved. This can initially be done with a soft-tipped wire (e.g. Glidewire, Terumo, Sunrise, FL, USA) under fluoroscopic imaging. This wire should be exchanged over a soft catheter for a stiff guidewire (e.g. Lunderquist and Amplatz), which should be placed in the distal thoracic aorta. One must ensure that these wires are not withdrawn or advanced during the procedure. Repositioning of a stiff guidewire without fluoroscopic guidance can result inadvertent cannulation of an arch vessel or aortic valve, aortic plaque or thrombus disruption, or aortic dissection.

Once stiff wire access is established via one femoral sheath, a pigtail catheter with radiopaque markers can be advanced over a soft wire in the contralateral sheath. If there is question about possible iliac occlusive disease that requires pre-procedure treatment, or if there is concern regarding aneurysmal anatomy (aortic length, renal artery location), angiography and intervention can be performed at this time.

Step 4. Delivery and Deployment

Main Body

Graft Orientation

Prior to insertion, the contralateral gate should be oriented under fluoroscopy. Typically, this involves maintaining orientation based on fluoroscopic graft markers to ensure the gate opens aligned with the contralateral common iliac to facilitate cannulation. The decision to cross the graft limbs is an exception to this orientation. This decision is sometimes guided on initial wire access with splayed bifurcations. If the wires appear to sit crossed low in the aneurysm, the operator should consider crossing the limbs in order to limit endotension, especially in shorter body devices such as the Gore Excluder. For longer body devices like the Cook Zenith, which have the contralateral gate closer to the bifurcation, such a maneuver is less optimal.

With orientation confirmed the device should be advanced slowly under fluoroscopy to confirm that positioning is maintained. Any rotation to the graft should be performed while the graft is being advanced to avoid building up unnecessary torque in the device. Care should also be taken to avoid rotating the graft within the proximal neck due to risk of embolic events from aortic thrombus. If there is a large thrombus burden, consider systemic heparinization prior to graft or wire insertion.

If insertion of the endograft device proves difficult, due to tortuous iliacs or distal aorta, there are several troubleshooting options available. The contralateral wire can be exchanged to a stiffer wire to take out any residual tension in the aneurysm or aortic bifurcation. A "buddy wire" of a second stiff wire can also be advanced up the ipsilateral system, to further straighten any tortuous segment.

Proximal Landing Zone

Once the endograft is sufficiently advanced, and both contralateral gate position and appropriate gantry angulation have been set, initial diagnostic imaging can be obtained. The use of a contrast injector is required for adequate opacification of visceral vessels. We prefer an initial angiogram with a high rate and small volume of contrast, typically 20 ml/s with a total volume of 20 ml of full-strength contrast. This should ensure visualization of both renal arteries.

With the ostium of the renal arteries marked on screen and the fluoroscopy table locked, initial deployment of the graft can begin. Initial deployment should begin *above* the target position, as many grafts tend to shift or "jump" distally (Figure 5.3). This also allows for the graft to be pulled down slowly during deployment, to a level just below the renal artery. Depending on the device, advancing

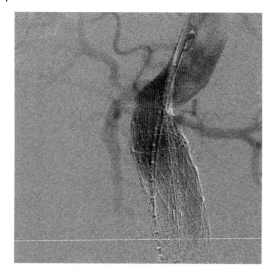

Figure 5.3 Repeat contrast angiography prior to complete deployment of the main body endograft can ensure placement of the covered stent just below the level of the lowest renal artery. The above picture demonstrates filling of the left renal artery with the proximal graft partially deployed.

the graft if it is positioned too low can prove difficult. Some grafts, such as the Excluder, have a repositionable proximal stent, which can be reconstrained within the sheath by the operator to ensure accurate deployment. The goal should be to place the graft within 0–2 mm of the caudal edge of the lowest renal. Maximal overlap will mitigate the risk of further aneurysmal degeneration, graft migration, or type I endoleak. It is important to know graft specifics, as different grafts will have fabric located at varying distances from the proximal stent.

After the proximal landing zone is established, the endograft is further deployed until the contralateral gate is deployed. At this point devices with suprarenal bare stents can now be deployed to set the proximal landing zone in place before gate cannulation and limb deployment.

Contralateral Gate Cannulation

For modular devices, the contralateral gate must be cannulated prior to completion of the main body deployment. This is however not the case in unibody devices such as the AFX™ graft (Endologix, Irvine, CA, USA). Several steps may assist the operator during main body deployment: orientation of the gate slightly anterior facilitates an easier angle of retrograde cannulation from the ipsilateral iliac sheath, balleting or crossing the limbs, and placement of the ipsilateral main body limb up the more tortuous iliac side (Figure 5.4).

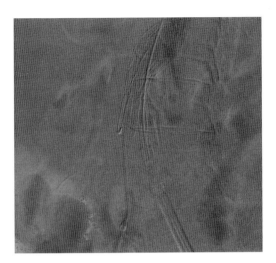

Figure 5.4 Cannulation of the contralateral gate can prove challenging, as demonstrated by the still image above. Operators must be facile with multiple catheters of various orientations to help ensure success.

Mostly dependent on catheter time and the experience of the operator, the following is an incomplete list of tips and tricks to assist with cannulation:

i) The use of a steerable hydrophile angled wire (e.g. angled Glidewire) with an appropriately angled catheter (e.g. Kumpe [Cook], Berenstein [Angiodynamic], or Sos 1/2 [Cook]).

ii) Frequent adjustment of the imaging gantry, both oblique and cephalad/caudal, to attempt to "open" the gate on fluoroscopic views.

iii) Placement of a stiff buddy wire through the contralateral sheath into the thoracic aorta to help guide the catheter and wire toward the contralateral gate.

iv) Advancement of a smaller French sheath into the aneurysm sac in conjunction with an angled catheter, which can be partially retracted into the sheath to allow for greater catheter-tip "steerability" (the "turret technique" [18]).

Gate cannulation is usually confirmed with the combination of contrast angiography and the ability to spin a pigtail catheter freely in the proximal neck of the graft.

If retrograde cannulation is not possible, antegrade cannulation can be attempted. Vascular access can be obtained via the axillary, brachial, or radial artery to allow for cannulation through the proximal graft body. The wire can then be snared from the iliac and exchanged for a stiffer wire, allowing for retrograde deployment. It is also possible to go "up-and-over" from the contralateral side, although this technique has a higher degree of difficulty depending on the device flow divider position.

If all above attempts fail, the final bailout maneuver is conversion of the bifurcated graft into an aorto-uni-iliac configuration, either by stacking aortic endocuffs or placement of a second main body endograft with the contralateral gate in the opposite orientation. In either case, the contralateral limb must be occluded, and a femoral-femoral bypass must be performed to reestablish limb perfusion.

Limb Deployment

Following cannulation of the contralateral gate, the contralateral iliac artery is evaluated with retrograde angiography through the femoral sheath. This should be performed under contralateral obliquity with a marker pigtail catheter to best visualize the iliac bifurcation and allow for accurate measurement of the length of limb needed. Most devices require at least 1–2 cm of iliac artery overlap for successful seal. Following measurement and deployment of the contralateral limb, similar measurements should be taken on the ipsilateral side following deployment of the remainder of the main body. If required, an ipsilateral extension can be used to aneurysmal iliac disease.

In patients with residual stenosis or kinking of the iliac limbs, aggressive angioplasty with a semicompliant balloon (e.g. Coda, Reliant, etc.) should be performed. For any recalcitrant lesions, consideration should be taken to deployment of a self-expanding bare-metal stent within the endograft. If the lesion is at the aortic bifurcation causing iliac compression, consider placement of kissing balloon-expandable stents.

Following deployment of the graft body and limbs, a semicompliant molding balloon should be used at the aortic neck, iliac gates, graft overlap, and distal iliac limbs to optimize seal. Angioplasty should not be performed outside of the graft as vessel rupture can occur.

Completion Angiogram

Following deployment and balloon angioplasty of the main body graft and iliac limbs, completion aortogram should be performed through a pigtail catheter placed above the renal arteries. In addition, any stiff wires should be removed prior to completion angiogram to allow the graft to sit in a more "natural" position. Using a contrast injector, we again opt for a high rate but with a higher volume of contrast to adequately evaluate for renal filling and any type I or II early or late endoleaks (Figure 5.5). As device sheaths are usually occlusive, it is also good practice to aspirate using 20 ml syringes to allow for contrast flow through the iliofemoral system.

Completion angiography should confirm the following:

i) Patency of both renal and hypogastric arteries
ii) Placement of the graft body adjacent to, ideally within 2 mm of, the lowest renal artery

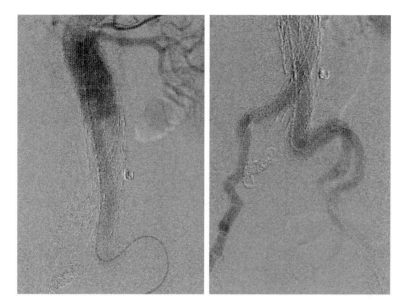

Figure 5.5 The completion angiogram above from a single case demonstrates excellent aneurysmal exclusion. The left renal artery is filling briskly (right) without evidence of Type I endoleak. The aneurysm does not fill early or late in the contrast run. And the bilateral iliac arteries fill and empty without evidence of Type IB or III endoleak (right hypogastric artery coiled).

iii) Adequately treated occlusive iliac disease
iv) Assess for early or late type I or II endoleaks

Step 5. Troubleshooting

Endoleaks

Should the completion angiography be concerning for a type I or III endoleak, these should be addressed immediately (Figure 5.6). The first step for nearly all endoleaks is to attempt balloon angioplasty. For type IA (proximal) leaks, this alone should be done if the distance between the lowest renal artery and the endograft is less than 3 mm. If this distance is greater than 5 mm, a proximal aortic cuff may be placed. This should then be balloon angioplastied as well. If a type IA leak persists despite these interventions, one may consider the placement of a Palmaz stent or an endovascular anchoring device. There are multiple systems currently available for this purpose. Similar to type IA, persistent type IB leaks may be

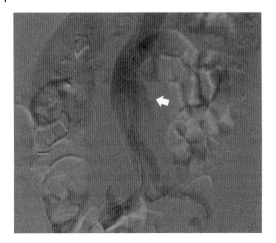

Figure 5.6 Completion angiogram demonstrates a Type IA endoleak. Aneurysmal sac filling is early and brisk in the contrast run, usually signifying leak around the proximal fixation stents.

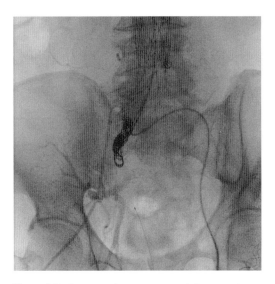

Figure 5.7 In cases where aneurysmal degeneration extends to the iliac arteries, hypogastric coiling allows for extension of graft coverage beyond the iliac bifurcation while minimizing the risk of endoleak.

remedied with a limb extension cuff. Type III leaks usually resolve with angioplasty provided there is enough component overlap. If this is not the case, bridging components may be introduced.

Type II endoleaks generally present long after the patient has left the angiography suite. These leaks can be detected on thin cut CTA, but angiography remains the gold standard for identifying the contributing vessel or vessels. It is also imperative to confirm that there is no concurrent type I or III leak. Aneurysmal sac enlargement greater than 5 mm is the generally accepted indication for intervention. The underlying principle for treatment of type II leaks is occlusion of the feeding artery. There are several accepted ways to accomplish this, including embolization, clipping, or surgical ligation. One should attempt to occlude the vessel as centrally as possible, as the development of collaterals may lead to eventual recurrence (Figure 5.7).

Inadvertent Coverage of Renal Arteries

Great care is taken to ensure the endograft is positioned appropriately below the renal arteries as not to accidentally cover one or, much worse, both after deployment. Should this occur, there are various maneuvers one may employ. The first two strategies involve attempting to displace the graft caudally using either a wire or a large balloon. Both are potentially very dangerous as aortic injury may occur. Preferably, one may place a stent in the affected renal artery. In some cases, the artery may need to be cannulated from a brachial approach. Surgical extra-anatomic bypass may be necessary should these efforts fail.

Should one encounter renal artery stenosis, this may be addressed following deployment of the aortic graft or at a later time. In some instances, stenosis may be discovered during preoperative planning and should the patient have severe renal insufficiency or hypertension, the surgeon may elect to stent the affected artery prior to performing the EVAR. One should be mindful that the stent may be dislodged or damaged at the time of graft deployment.

Iliac Artery Considerations

Depending on the anatomy of the common iliac artery, extension into the external iliac may be required. In this instance, it is important to remember to address the hypogastric in hopes of preventing a future type II endoleak. One may either embolize the hypogastric or attempt to preserve flow through a branched graft, stent placement, or open bypass from the external.

Conclusion

EVAR is now universally accepted as the first-line treatment for AAA in patients who meet the anatomic criteria for stent-graft placement. Careful preoperative planning and technical considerations are essential to a successful outcome of this procedure.

References

1 Volodos, N.L., Shekhanin, V.E., Karpovich, I.P. et al. (1986). A self-fixing synthetic blood vessel endoprosthesis. *Vestn. Khir. Im. I I Grek.* 137 (11): 123–125.

2 Greenhalgh, R.M., Brown, L.C., Kwong, G.P. et al. (2004). Comparison of endovascular aneurysm repair with open repair in patients with abdominal aortic aneurysm (EVAR trial 1), 30-day operative mortality results: randomised controlled trial. *Lancet* 364 (9437): 843–848.

3 Prinssen, M., Verhoeven, E.L., Buth, J. et al. (2004). A randomized trial comparing conventional and endovascular repair of abdominal aortic aneurysms. *N. Engl. J. Med.* 351 (16): 1607–1618.

4 Lederle, F.A., Freischlag, J.A., Kyriakides, T.C. et al. (2009). Outcomes following endovascular vs open repair of abdominal aortic aneurysm: a randomized trial. *JAMA* 302 (14): 1535–1542.

5 Torella, F. (2004). Effect of improved endograft design on outcome of endovascular aneurysm repair. *J. Vasc. Surg.* 40 (2): 216–221.

6 De Bruin, J.L., Baas, A.F., Buth, J. et al. (2010). Long-term outcome of open or endovascular repair of abdominal aortic aneurysm. *N. Engl. J. Med.* 362 (20): 1881–1889.

7 Franks, S.C., Sutton, A.J., Bown, M.J., and Sayers, R.D. (2007). Systematic review and meta-analysis of 12 years of endovascular abdominal aortic aneurysm repair. *Eur. J. Vasc. Endovasc. Surg.* 33 (2): 154–171.

8 Paravastu, S.C., Jayarajasingam, R., Cottam, R. et al. (2014). Endovascular repair of abdominal aortic aneurysm. *Cochrane Database Syst. Rev.* (1): CD004178.

9 United Kingdom ETI, Greenhalgh, R.M., Brown, L.C. et al. (2010). Endovascular repair of aortic aneurysm in patients physically ineligible for open repair. *N. Engl. J. Med.* 362 (20): 1872–1880.

10 Joels, C.S., Langan, E.M. 3rd, Daley, C.A. et al. (2009). Changing indications and outcomes for open abdominal aortic aneurysm repair since the advent of endovascular repair. *Am. Surg.* 75 (8): 665–669; discussion 9–70.

11 Aburahma, A.F., Campbell, J.E., Mousa, A.Y. et al. (2011). Clinical outcomes for hostile versus favorable aortic neck anatomy in endovascular aortic aneurysm repair using modular devices. *J. Vasc. Surg.* 54 (1): 13–21.

12 Wyss, T.R., Dick, F., Brown, L.C., and Greenhalgh, R.M. (2011). The influence of thrombus, calcification, angulation, and tortuosity of attachment sites on the time to the first graft-related complication after endovascular aneurysm repair. *J. Vasc. Surg.* 54 (4): 965–971.

13 Sharafuddin, M.J. and Marjan, A.E. (2017). Current status of carbon dioxide angiography. *J. Vasc. Surg.* 66 (2): 618–637.

14 Hoshina, K., Kato, M., Miyahara, T. et al. (2010). A retrospective study of intravascular ultrasound use in patients undergoing endovascular aneurysm repair: its usefulness and a description of the procedure. *Eur. J. Vasc. Endovasc. Surg.* 40 (5): 559–563.

15 Kauvar, D.S., Martin, E.D., and Givens, M.D. (2016). Thirty-day outcomes after elective percutaneous or open endovascular repair of abdominal aortic aneurysms. *Ann. Vasc. Surg.* 31: 46–51.

16 Vierhout, B.P., Pol, R.A., Ott, M.A. et al. (2019). Randomized multicenter trial on percutaneous versus open access in endovascular aneurys repair (PiERO). *J. Vasc. Surg.* 69 (5): 1429–1436.

17 Swinnen, J., Chao, A., Tiwari, A. et al. (2010). Vertical or transverse incisions for access to the femoral artery: a randomized control study. *Ann. Vasc. Surg.* 24 (3): 336–341.

18 Kahn, S.L., Arslan, B., and Masrani, A. (2018). *Interventional and Endovascular Tips and Tricks of the Trade*, The Turret Technique for Contralateral Gate Access. Oxford University Press.

6

Severe Renal Artery Stenosis

How to Intervene

Mohammad Hashim Mustehsan[1], Cristina Sanina[2], and Jose D. Tafur[3]

[1] Division of Cardiology, Albert Einstein College of Medicine-Montefiore Medical Center, Bronx, NY, USA
[2] Division of Cardiology, Department of Medicine, Beth Israel Deaconess Medical Center, Harvard Medical School, Boston, MA, USA
[3] Department of Cardiovascular Diseases, John Ochsner Heart & Vascular Institute, The Ochsner Clinical School, University of Queensland School of Medicine, New Orleans, LA, USA

Introduction

Renal artery stenosis (RAS) is most frequently secondary to atherosclerotic renal artery stenosis (ARAS) (90%). Fibromuscular dysplasia (FMD) accounts for most of the remaining cases. Clinical manifestations include severe and refractory hypertension, ischemic nephropathy, and cardiac destabilizing syndromes (flash-pulmonary edema, heart failure, acute coronary syndrome). Patients should be tested for RAS if they have: early (age ≤30 years) or late (age ≥55 years) onset of hypertension, resistant, accelerated, or malignant hypertension, acute renal failure after initiation of ACEi/ARB, renal atrophy, or sudden, unexplained pulmonary edema. Screening for RAS is performed using noninvasive imaging, namely renal artery Doppler ultrasound, computer tomographic angiography (CTA), or magnetic resonance angiography (MRA). Invasive testing with digital subtraction angiography is still considered the gold standard but carries the risk of procedural complications. Evidence from RCTs has failed to demonstrate a benefit for revascularization compared to medical therapy as an initial approach. However, revascularization for cases refractory to medical therapy is still indicated and appropriate patient selection is essential.

Endovascular Interventions: A Step-by-Step Approach, First Edition. Edited by Jose M. Wiley, Cristina Sanina, George D. Dangas, and Prakash Krishnan.
© 2023 John Wiley & Sons Ltd. Published 2023 by John Wiley & Sons Ltd.

Patients with recurrent flash-pulmonary edema, hemodynamically significant RAS, refractory ACS, refractory hypertension resistant to optimal medical therapy, or progressively worsening renal insufficiency should be considered for RAS revascularization. The main goal of RAS revascularization is to prevent progression of, and potentially reverse, complications of RAS including hypertension, cardiac destabilizing syndromes, and ischemic nephropathy.

Strategies to maximize results and prevent short- and long-term complications include radial access, no-touch techniques, and intravascular imaging. After intervention, all patients should be placed on at least single-antiplatelet therapy with aspirin. Ensure close outpatient follow-up, along with postprocedural renal Doppler ultrasound at 1, 6, and 12 months, and annually thereafter.

Background and Clinical Significance

Epidemiology

Renal artery stenosis (RAS) is defined as an abnormal narrowing of one or both renal arteries. While there are several potential etiologies of RAS (Table 6.1), the overwhelming majority (~90%) of cases can be attributed to ARAS – with FMD accounting for most of the remaining cases (~10%), typically in younger females [1]. ARAS is common and its prevalence depends on the population being screened, with incidence increasing with age, affecting both men and women equally. ARAS is present in about 7% of patients over the age of 65 years and is more prevalent (~60%) in patients with hypertension, atherosclerotic arterial disease, and renal insufficiency [2].

Clinical Manifestations

Clinical manifestations of RAS include hypertension, ischemic nephropathy, and cardiac destabilizing syndromes.

Table 6.1 Etiologies of renal artery stenosis.

Atherosclerotic renal artery stenosis (ARAS) – 90% of cases

Fibromuscular dysplasia (FMD) – ~10% of cases

Trauma with resulting dissection

Renal artery dissection

Congenital

Williams syndrome (genetic condition, thought to involve deletion of the Elastin gene)

Hypertension: Both unilateral and bilateral RAS can lead to hypertension, but by slightly different mechanisms. It is posited that hemodynamically significant unilateral RAS results in the activation of the renin-angiotensin-aldosterone system (RAAS), leading to increased arterial tone and hypertension. Due to the preserved function of the contralateral kidney, appropriate natriuresis continues to occur, and no significant volume overload exists. Bilateral RAS similarly leads to RAAS activation; however, there is significant concomitant volume overload given that neither kidney can accommodate compensatory natriuresis. RAS-related hypertension is the leading cause of secondary hypertension and may be difficult to control.

Ischemic nephropathy: Hemodynamically significant RAS can result in ischemic nephropathy, which is characterized by loss of renal mass, reduction in glomerular filtration, and renal parenchymal fibrosis. Clinically this presents as progressive loss of renal function, proteinuria, and renal atrophy.

Cardiac destabilizing syndromes: RAS-related volume overload and hypertension can lead to flash-pulmonary edema (particularly in the absence of valvular disease or heart failure), acute coronary syndrome, and refractory heart failure [3].

Patient Selection: Who to Screen for RAS

There are no existing guidelines on routine screening for RAS, and screening can be initiated by clinicians based on patient presentation and risk factors. Currently, Class I recommendations for screening by the ACC/AHA guidelines [4] include early (age ≤ 30 years) or late (age ≥ 55 years) onset of hypertension, resistant (hypertension with systolic blood pressure $\geq 140 \pm$ diastolic blood pressure ≥ 90 despite use of three or more oral agents including a diuretic), accelerated (sudden worsening of previously controlled hypertension) or malignant (severe hypertension with evidence of end-organ damage) hypertension, acute renal failure after initiation of ACEi/ARB, renal atrophy, asymmetric renal dimensions (discrepancy of >1.5 cm), and sudden, unexplained pulmonary edema. Other indications for screening include unexplained renal failure, new dialysis initiation, vascular disease (coronary disease or peripheral arterial disease), and unexplained heart failure [4] (Table 6.2).

RAS Assessment

Noninvasive RAS Assessment

Renal doppler ultrasound (DUS): Renal DUS is an excellent initial test for the assessment of RAS, given that it is low cost and noninvasive nature. Peak systolic velocity (PSV) >200 cm/s by Doppler is 95% sensitive and 90% specific for

Table 6.2 Who to screen for RAS (AHA/ACC 2006).

Clinical scenario	Indication class	Level of evidence
Hypertension onset: early (age ≤30 years) or late (age ≥55 years)	Class I	LOE B
Accelerated, resistant, or malignant hypertension	Class I	LOE C
New azotemia or renal dysfunction after ACEi/ARB use	Class I	LOE B
Unexplained atrophic kidney or size discrepancy between kidneys of >1.5 cm	Class I	LOE B
Sudden, unexplained pulmonary edema	Class I	LOE B
Unexplained renal dysfunction/new dialysis initiation	Class IIa	LOE B
Multivessel coronary artery disease	Class IIb	LOE B
Unexplained congestive heart failure	Class IIb	LOE C
Refractory angina	Class IIb	LOE C

Source: Hirsch et al. [4]/American Heart Association.

identifying a renal artery lesion >50%, while an end-diastolic velocity of >150 cm/s is highly predictive of a severe (>80%) lesion [5]. Additional diagnostic criteria include a renal artery PSV to aortic PSV ratio >3.5, rise time >0.07 seconds, acceleration index <300 cm/s, and a difference in renal resistive index >0.15. It is important to note that after renal artery revascularization, DUS velocities are increased due to a loss of arterial compliance – which can lead to overestimation of in-stent restenosis (ISR). Postintervention a PSV >395 cm/s is most predictive of significant (>70%) ISR [5]. Factors that decrease the diagnostic yield of DUS include patient body habitus, bowel gas, and sonographer skills.

Computer tomographic angiography (CTA): CTA has been shown to have a sensitivity of up to 96% and a specificity of up to 99% for diagnosing significant (>50% stenosis) RAS [6]. CTA can not only provide high-resolution images of the renal arteries but can also be used to generate three-dimensional (3D) angiograms of the aorta, accessory, and visceral arteries. CTA can be used for follow-up imaging after renal artery intervention since image quality is not limited by the presence of a stent (in contrast to MRA). A significant limitation of CTA is the necessity of using a high volume (100–150 cc) of iodinated contrast, making it an unattractive diagnostic modality in patients with renal dysfunction.

Magnetic resonance angiography (MRA): MRA also has a very high sensitivity (90–100%) and specificity (~94%) for detection of significant RAS. Like CTA, MRA can provide high-resolution reconstructions of the aorta, renal, and visceral arteries. The use of gadolinium as a contrast agent, which is less nephrotoxic than iodinated contrast agents, gives MRA an advantage over CTA. However, in end-stage renal disease (GFR $<30\,ml/min/1.73\,m^2$), gadolinium carries a risk of nephrogenic systemic fibrosis. Furthermore, MRA provides suboptimal images for follow-up of RAS postintervention due to significant streak artifacts from stents [7].

Invasive RAS Assessment

Digital subtraction angiography (DSA): DSA is a 2D imaging modality which is still considered the gold standard in the RAS diagnosis. However, due to its invasive nature, it is only performed if noninvasive testing is unrevealing, or a concomitant angiographic procedure is being performed. An RAS of >70% is considered significant, while a moderate lesion (50–70%) requires testing for hemodynamic significance. A lesion is considered hemodynamically significant if there is resting translesional systolic gradient of $\geq20\,mmHg$, a mean translesional gradient of $\geq10\,mmHg$, or a renal fractional flow reserve (RFFR) ≤0.8 [3]. Limitations of DSA include risks associated with vascular access, contrast nephropathy, risk of plaque embolization, and radiation exposure [7].

Indications for Revascularization

The goal of revascularization of RAS is to prevent progression of, and potentially reverse, complications of RAS including hypertension, cardiac destabilizing syndromes, and ischemic nephropathy. Multiple randomized controlled clinical trials have failed to demonstrate a significant difference between revascularization and medical therapy in the management of hypertension [8–10]. The "Stent Placement in Patients with Atherosclerotic Renal Artery Stenosis and Impaired Renal Function: A Randomized Trial (STAR)" study enrolled 140 patients with RAS (>50%) and renal dysfunction (GFR <80) and compared outcomes with medical therapy versus medical therapy and renal revascularization. There were no significant differences between the groups; however, 30% of the patients in the revascularization arm had no significant RAS (<70%) and were not candidates for renal artery revascularization [8]. The "Angioplasty and Stenting for Renal Artery Lesions (ASTRAL)" trial also did not show a benefit of revascularization over medical therapy. The trial, however, had limitation as only 60% of the patients had significant RAS and the revascularization group required fewer antihypertensive medications (making direct comparison difficult with the medical therapy only group) [9]. Finally, the "Stenting and Medical Therapy for Atherosclerotic Renal Artery Stenosis (CORAL)" trial assessed the utility of revascularization for RAS in patients with hypertension (defined as systolic blood pressure $\geq155\,mmHg$ on ≥2

antihypertensive medications), RAS ($\geq$70% stenosis), and chronic kidney disease (CKD) (GFR <60). The CORAL trial also found no benefit for RAS revascularization compared to medical therapy alone – however, this trial was limited by a lack of functional assessment for RAS and the fact that patients in both arms had improvement in blood pressure (suggesting poor blood pressure control at baseline) [10].

Given trial results and limitations, there is still a role for revascularization for RAS in patients with poorly controlled hypertension on optimal medical therapy (three or more agents, including a diuretic), patients with recurrent flash-pulmonary edema and those with progressive renal dysfunction [3].

Based on the ACC/AHA guidelines, the following patient profiles are most likely to benefit from revascularization for RAS: patients with recurrent flash-pulmonary edema (Class I, LOE B), patients with hemodynamically significant RAS and refractory acute coronary syndrome (Class IIa, LOE B), patients with refractory hypertension who cannot tolerate or fail medical therapy (Class IIa, LOE B), patients with progressive CKD (Class IIa, LOE B), and patient with unilateral RAS (Class IIb, LOE C) [4] (Table 6.3).

Revascularization is not indicated in patients who are asymptomatic, when RAS is not thought to be the causative etiology of symptoms, patients with uncontrolled hypertension not on optimal medical therapy (three or more agents, including a diuretic) and patients with CKD III or greater with renal atrophy (kidney pole-to-pole size $\leq$7 cm), and patients on hemodialysis for $\geq$3 months [3].

Table 6.3 Indications for renal artery revascularization (AHA/ACC 2006).

Clinical scenario	Recommendation class/level of evidence
Cardiac destabilizing syndromes with severe RAS or moderate RAS with mean translesional gradient of $\geq$10 mmHg	Class I/LOE B
CKD IV with bilateral moderate RAS with mean translesional gradient of $\geq$10 mmHg and kidney size >7 cm	Class IIa/LOE B
CKD IV with global renal ischemia	Class IIb/LOE B
Resistant hypertension and severe RAS	Class IIa/LOE B
Recurrent heart failure with unilateral moderate RAS with mean translesional gradient of $\geq$10 mmHg	Class I/LOE B
Resistant hypertension and severe unilateral RAS	Class IIa/LOE B

Source: Hirsch et al. [4]/American Heart Association.

Intervention

Step 1. Vascular access

Place the patient on operative table in supine position. Appropriately prep and drape the access site. Traditionally, renal artery interventions are performed via femoral access; however, radial access (either radial artery can be used, however, left one may be a shorter distance to the renal arteries) has shown a lower risk for vascular-related complications [3]. When using radial access, it is important to consider the height of the patient appropriate length of equipment (use 125-cm long guiding catheters with 150-cm balloon or stent shafts) to reach the renal arteries with adequate guide catheter support [11]. Once access is obtained (typically 6 Fr sheath), the patient should be heparinized to achieve an activated clotting time (ACT) ≥ 200 seconds – which should be maintained throughout the procedure.

Step 2. Diagnostic aortogram

Advance a 0.035-in. guidewire to the T12-L1 level, with a goal to be slightly proximal to the origin of the renal arteries (typically at L1). Using a pigtail catheter, obtain an aortogram with about 10 cc of contrast to delineate the origin of the renal arteries (optimal views: LAO 20 for right renal artery, RAO 20 for left renal artery) – unless a CTA or MRA was already performed.

Step 3. Engagement of renal artery

The renal artery of choice can be engaged with either the "no-touch" technique, "telescoping" technique or with Direct engagement: a diagnostic soft catheter (MP or JR4 from radial access or IMA, JR4, renal standard curve from femoral approach) is gently manipulated to be seated at the ostium of the renal artery. This approach is not recommended with interventional guides as it carries a higher risk for dissection and embolization.

No-touch technique: deploy a 0.035-in. J-wire in the aorta, gently advance a guide catheter toward the target renal artery. When the guide catheter approaches the renal artery, insert an angioplasty guidewire through the guide into the renal artery and past the target lesion. Then, gently withdraw the 0.035-in. J-wire.

Telescoping technique: insert a diagnostic catheter through a larger (typically 2 Fr larger) guide catheter. The two catheters are advanced over a 0.014-in. wire, and the ostium of the renal artery is engaged with the diagnostic catheter. The 0.014-in. wire is used to cross the lesion, and the guide catheter is advanced over the diagnostic catheter to engage the renal artery (Figure 6.1) [11].

Step 4. Diagnostic angiography

Once the guide catheter has been used to engage the renal artery, a selective diagnostic angiogram can be performed.

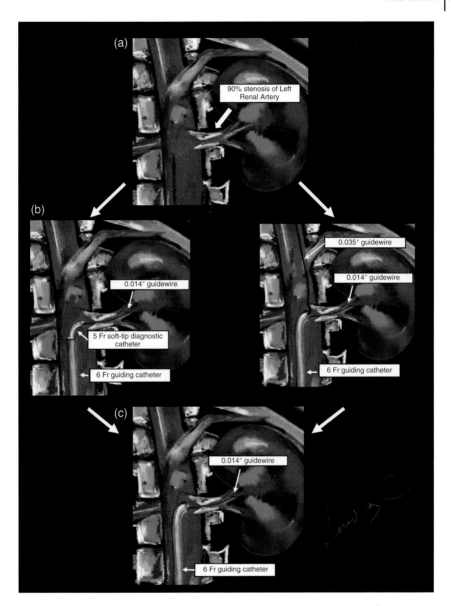

Figure 6.1 Indirect engagement of renal artery: (a) renal artery stenosis (b) "telescoping" technique and (c) "no-touch" technique. *Source:* Artist credit: Cristina Sanina.

Step 5. Renal artery intervention

Begin by dilating at the renal ostium prior to any subsequent distal inflations. The diameter of a predilated ostium or intravascular ultrasound (IVUS) can be used to guide stent sizing. Stent sizing is critically important in reducing risk of

ISR, along with benefits in blood pressure control [3]. The use of a premounted balloon-expandable bare-metal stent (BMS) is recommended [11]. Prior to stent deployment, there should be angiographic confirmation that the stent covers the renal artery ostium (confirm in anterior–posterior and RAO 20 [for left renal artery]/LAO 20 [for right renal artery] angulations). After stent deployment, perform a completion angiogram. This is to confirm renal artery flow, appropriate stent positioning, and expansion.

Step 6. Disengagement
   When the intervention is completed, disengage the guide catheter from the renal artery, while leaving the angioplasty wire in the vessel. After careful disengagement, the angioplasty wire can be slowly withdrawn from the renal artery. The introducer sheath can finally be removed once all wires and catheters are removed.

Step 7. Postprocedural management:
   Check distal pulses at the access site to ensure return to preprocedural baseline.
   After intervention, all patients should be placed on at least single-antiplatelet therapy with aspirin, given that the role of dual antiplatelet therapy after renal artery stenting is not yet established. If aspirin is contraindicated, clopidogrel can be used as an alternative.
   Ensure close outpatient follow-up, along with postprocedural renal DUS at 1, 6, and 12 months, and annually thereafter [12].
   Blood pressure should be monitored closely at postprocedural visits and antihypertensive medications adjusted per existing guidelines.

References

1 Slovut, D.P. and Olin, J.W. (2004). Fibromuscular dysplasia. *N. Engl. J. Med.* 350 (18): 1862–1871.
2 Hansen, K.J., Edwards, M.S., Craven, T.E. et al. (2002). Prevalence of renovascular disease in the elderly: a population-based study. *J. Vasc. Surg.* 36 (3): 443–451.
3 Prince, M., Tafur, J.D., and White, C.J. (2019). When and how should we revascularize patients with atherosclerotic renal artery stenosis? *J. Am. Coll. Cardiol. Intv.* 12 (6): 505–517.
4 Hirsch, A.T., Haskal, Z.J., Hertzer, N.R. et al. (2006). ACC/AHA 2005 practice guidelines for the management of patients with peripheral arterial disease (lower extremity, renal, mesenteric, and abdominal aortic). *Circulation* 113 (11).
5 Chi, Y.-W., White, C.J., Thornton, S., and Milani, R.V. (2009). Ultrasound velocity criteria for renal in-stent restenosis. *J. Vasc. Surg.* 50 (1): 119–123.

6 Kim, T.S., Chung, J.W., Park, J.H. et al. (1998). Renal artery evaluation: comparison of spiral CT angiography to intra-arterial DSA. *J. Vasc. Interv. Radiol.* 9 (4): 553–559.

7 Colyer, W.R., Eltahawy, E., and Cooper, C.J. (2011). Renal artery stenosis: optimizing diagnosis and treatment. *Prog. Cardiovasc. Dis.* 54 (1): 29–35.

8 Bax, L. (2009). Stent placement in patients with atherosclerotic renal artery stenosis and impaired renal function. *Ann. Intern. Med.* 150 (12): 840.

9 ASTRAL Investigators (2009). Revascularization versus medical therapy for renal-artery stenosis. *N. Engl. J. Med.* 361 (20): 1953–1962.

10 Cooper, C.J., Murphy, T.P., Cutlip, D.E. et al. (2014). Stenting and medical therapy for atherosclerotic renal-artery stenosis. *N. Engl. J. Med.* 370 (1): 13–22.

11 Safian, R.D. and Madder, R.D. (2009). Refining the approach to renal artery revascularization. *J. Am. Coll. Cardiol. Intv.* 2 (3): 161–174.

12 Tafur, J.D. and White, C.J. (2017). Renal artery stenosis: when to revascularize in 2017. *Curr. Probl. Cardiol.* 42 (4): 110–135.

7

Mesenteric Ischemia

Chronic and Acute Management

David A. Hirschl

Department of Radiology, Albert Einstein College of Medicine-Montefiore Medical Center, Bronx, NY, USA

Introduction

Acute and chronic mesenteric ischemia consist of a group of pathologic processes which compromise blood flow to the bowel. While chronic disease typically causes postprandial abdominal pain, acute occlusion of the mesenteric vasculature can be life-threatening. Advances in endovascular devices and techniques have led to a less invasive means of treatment compared with open revascularization. While surgery remains the therapy of choice in patients with peritonitis due to bowel necrosis, endovascular therapy has been shown to have a decreased in-hospital mortality for the treatment of mesenteric ischemia. This chapter will discuss the diagnosis and management of acute and chronic mesenteric ischemia with attention to endovascular therapeutic interventions.

Chronic Mesenteric Ischemia

The most common cause of chronic mesenteric ischemia (CMI) is an arterial occlusive disease with atherosclerosis accounting for 35–75% of cases [1]. Other causes include vasculitis, fibromuscular dysplasia, segmental arterial mediolysis, and median arcuate ligament syndrome [2]. CMI is most prevalent in older people, and women are three times more likely to develop CMI compared to men [3].

Endovascular Interventions: A Step-by-Step Approach, First Edition. Edited by Jose M. Wiley, Cristina Sanina, George D. Dangas, and Prakash Krishnan.
© 2023 John Wiley & Sons Ltd. Published 2023 by John Wiley & Sons Ltd.

The most common site is the proximal superior mesenteric artery (SMA). Due to extensive collateral flow in the bowel, CMI usually presents if two of the three visceral arteries are involved. If the patient has undergone prior bowel or aortic surgery, a collateral flow may have been disrupted which increases the risk of CMI due to single-vessel disease [4, 5]. The goal of therapy is to restore flow to the bowel. Surgical intervention has previously been considered the gold standard of therapy. Currently, endovascular intervention has gained favor in the treatment of this disease process by drastically reducing perioperative morbidity. Studies have also shown the in-hospital mortality rate following endovascular intervention to be 3.7% compared to 13% for surgical intervention [6]; however, long-term mortality is similar [7]. Multiple societies including The American College of Radiology recommend an "Endovascular First" approach to treatment [8]. Successful recanalization of a severely diseased vessel or chronic total occlusion (CTO) requires a planned approach with consideration to anatomy, planned access site, and equipment. A careful review of preprocedure imaging, preferably a high-quality computed tomography angiography (CTA) will allow the operator to make adequate preprocedural decisions thereby improving technical success rates. Current guidelines advocate primary stenting as the preferred method of endovascular revascularization. Primary stenting has higher postprocedural patency rate compared with angioplasty alone due to elastic recoil [9–13]. The indications for endovascular intervention are listed in Table 7.1.

Step 1. Vascular Access and Sheath Selection

Most commonly, access for mesenteric artery intervention is gained through a common femoral artery approach. An alternate approach is through the left brachial artery; however, this is associated with a higher rate of access site complications [14]. More recently, the radial approach has been used. After puncturing the

Table 7.1 Indications for percutaneous intervention.

1) Symptomatic patients with clinical triad:
   a) Unintentional weight loss
   b) Postprandial abdominal pain and/or food aversion
   c) Two-vessel disease on imaging
2) Symptomatic patients with aortic dissection or spontaneous mesenteric artery dissection causing compromised mesenteric perfusion as a result of the involvement of at least two of the three visceral arteries
3) As part of a repair in a patient undergoing abdominal aortic aneurysm repair (EVAR)

Source: Adapted from Pillai et al. [2].

chosen vessel, a vascular sheath is placed. The size and length of the sheath will be determined by the devices intended for use as well as access site. For femoral access many operators will select a 5–7 Fr vascular sheath ranging in length from 45 to 55 cm. Angled sheaths or guiding catheters will provide additional support for therapeutic devices. Larger sheath sizes will facilitate the use of guiding catheter for increased support in a coaxial system. Tip deflecting access sheaths, guide catheter such as the Morph AccessPro, and Universal Deflectable guides (Biocardia, San Carlos, CA, USA), can be helpful in negotiating the challenging SMA angles when a femoral approach is chosen. The brachial approach, which can provide greater pushability and torquability for unfavorable SMA angles, requires a longer sheath, typically 90 cm.

Step 2. Diagnostic Angiography

A flush catheter is positioned in the abdominal aorta above the origin of the celiac artery. A lateral digital subtraction angiogram is performed to characterize the occlusion length in the SMA, the presence of a stump, calcifications, as well as to evaluate patency of the celiac artery [14] (Figure 7.1).

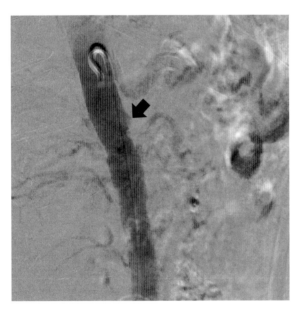

Figure 7.1 Flush aortagram performed via a femoral approach. Imaging is performed in a lateral view. Note the presence of a vascular stump at the expected location of the SMA (arrow).

Step 3. Vessel Selection

While working in a lateral view, the occluded vessel or stump is probed with a diagnostic catheter and hydrophilic wire such as a 0.035-in. Glidewire (Terumo, Elkton, MD, USA). Some diagnostic catheter choices include a C1, Simmons I, or Sos Omni Selective catheters (Angiodynamics, Latham, NY, USA). If a 0.035 wire cannot be advanced through a CTO, a guiding catheter can be introduced over the wire to provide additional support. If a 0.035 wire still cannot be advanced through the lesion, a 0.018 or a 0.014 wire can be used with an appropriately matched microcatheter (Figures 7.2 and 7.3).

Step 4. Selective Angiography

A catheter is advanced over the wire and through the lesion. A hydrophilic glide catheter (Terumo, Elkton, MD, USA) may be needed if the catheter cannot be easily advanced through the diseased vessel. Selective angiography of the SMA is performed through a diagnostic catheter or microcatheter to ensure the catheter tip is in the true lumen of the vessel and a dissection or perforation has not occurred. The angiogram will also determine the landing site of a stent. Intravascular pressure measurements can be made at this point. A gradient greater than 10 mmHg is considered significant.

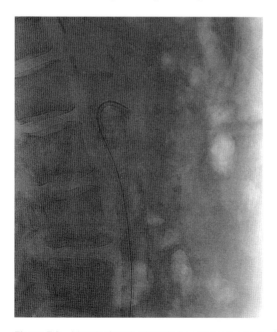

Figure 7.2 Morph sheath placed via a femoral approach. The tip of the sheath is at the ostium of a highly calcified superior mesenteric artery.

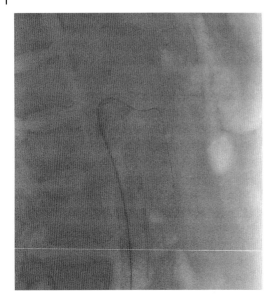

Figure 7.3 A hydrophilic wire has been advanced through a stenotic lesion using a Morph sheath as support.

Step 5. Placement of a Working Wire

A nonhydrophilic working wire is replaced in the SMA through the catheter. The wire should be positioned distal enough to have good purchase within the vessel, but not too distal in a branch vessel where it could cause a perforation. The catheter is exchanged over the wire for a stent or angioplasty balloon. Embolic prevention has been observed in selected patients when using an embolic protection device [15]. These devices are used as a working wire while having an embolic protection apparatus such as a filter or balloon occlusion at the distal end of the wire. If a 0.035 device is chosen for intervention, the second wire like a V-18 or V-14 ControlWire (Boston Scientific, Marlborough, MA, USA) can be used as a buddy wire for additional support. The vascular sheath or guiding catheter should be as close to the ostium of the vessel as possible to support passage of a balloon or stent.

Step 6. Stent Placement

A balloon-expandable stent is advanced over the wire and positioned in the proximal vessel. Before final positioning and deployment, an angiogram can be performed through the side arm of the sheath so that the proximal landing of the stent can be visualized. The proximal end of the stent should be deployed 3–5 mm extending into the aorta to ensure all proximal/ostial disease is covered.

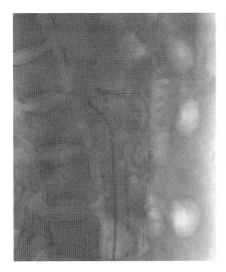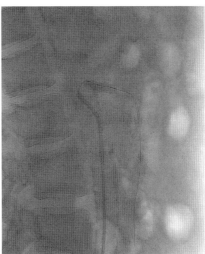

Figure 7.4 Balloon-expandable stent placement. Note minimal extension of the proximal aspect of the stent into the aorta.

Balloon-expandable stents are preferred over self-expanding stents due to the precise placement. Stent selection will be based on the target vessel size and length of disease. Typical stent dimensions range from 5 to 7 mm × 15 to 40 mm. An additional stent may be deployed if the initial stent does not fully cover the target lesion. A self-expanding stent can be used in more distal lesions or if an extension is required. Predilation using an angioplasty balloon may be needed if the stent cannot be advanced over the wire and through the lesion. Predilation can also be used if the vessel is completely occluded or the lesion is judged to be high grade. Predilation may increase the risk of distal thromboembolization (Figure 7.4).

Step 7. Posttreatment Angiography

A posttreatment angiogram is performed from the aorta. Residual stenosis of less than 30% is considered technically successful [14]. Intravascular pressure measurements can also be acquired with a gradient of less than 10 mmHg desired. Carefully evaluate the angiogram for evidence of distal embolization. Comparison with the prestent/angioplasty angiogram is essential (Figure 7.5).

Step 8. Revision

Poststent placement angioplasty or additional stenting may be necessary if the angiographic result is not adequate or if the pressure gradient is higher than 10 mmHg.

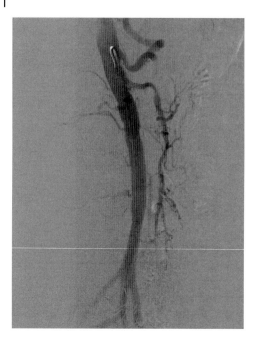

Figure 7.5 Poststent angiogram performed using a flush catheter via a femoral approach.

If present and recognized, distal embolization may require aspiration using an appropriately sized thrombectomy catheter. If the emboli cannot be aspirated, the patient is treated with anticoagulation. If signs of bowel infarction develop, emergent surgery with bowel resection is warranted.

Complications

The mortality rate for endovascular intervention is between 0% and 19% [2]. When compared to open surgical intervention, there is a nonstatistically significant decrease in 30-day mortality [7]. Morbidity rates for endovascular repair range from 0% to 31% [2]. The most common complications are related to the vascular access site and include hematoma, dissection, thrombosis, and distal thromboembolization. Thrombosis and distal embolization in the mesenteric artery resulting in acute bowel ischemia with the need for resection following endovascular intervention occur in 2–8% of patients [15–17]. Open surgical revascularization is associated with a higher rate of in-hospital complications including bowel resection and infection [7].

Lesion characteristics which have been shown to increase the risk of distal embolization include recanalization of a CTO, and lesion length greater than 2 cm. Subacute symptoms (two to four weeks) have also been shown to increase risk of embolization [15]. Of the rare periprocedural mortalities that occur after endovascular intervention, 50–60% of cases are related to distal embolization [18, 19].

Follow-Up and Outcomes

Patients should be placed on dual antiplatelet therapy such as clopidogrel and aspirin (81 or 235 mg). On the day of the procedure, a loading dose of clopidogrel 300 mg is given followed by 75 mg daily for at least one month [14]. Other authors advocate for 3–12 months clopidogrel therapy [9, 16]. Doppler evaluation biannually during the first year and annually thereafter has been suggested; however, no consensus guidelines exist. Velocities of >70% of peak systolic velocities of 412–445 cm/s in the SMA and 289–363 cm/s in the celiac artery suggest in-stent restenosis [2]. Such findings may warrant angiography and endovascular revision. Technical success rates of endovascular stent placement range from 85 to 100%, with lower rates for angioplasty alone [2]. Primary patency of bare-metal stents ranges from 58 to 88% in the first year and 30 to 81% in the third year [10–13, 20–24].

Acute Mesenteric Ischemia

Acute mesenteric ischemia (AMI) encompasses a variety of pathologies that interrupt blood flow to the small bowel resulting in ischemia, inflammation, and possible necrosis. If not promptly recognized, mortality rates approach 50–80% [25–27]. Etiologies include nonocclusive mesenteric ischemia (NOMI), and occlusive disease which may be due to thromboembolism (50%), mesenteric arterial thrombosis (15–25%), or mesenteric venous thrombosis (5–15%) [28, 29].

Approximately 50% of all AMI cases are due to acute mesenteric artery embolism [30, 31]. The origin of thrombus is most often cardiogenic in the setting of atrial fibrillation, severe left ventricular dysfunction, or endocarditis. Cholesterol emboli may also come from the aorta. Emboli will typically lodge 3–10 cm from the SMA origin and may spare proximal branch vessels supplying the proximal jejunum and the mid colic artery. After diagnosing acute embolic disease in the SMA, a thorough review of the imaging is necessary to evaluate for concurrent emboli in other vascular beds which can occur in over 20% of cases [30].

Unlike acute embolic disease, patients with AMI related to arterial thrombosis usually occlude the vessel at the origin. Most often this occurs in the setting of underlying atherosclerotic plaque. Review of the patient's history may reveal evidence of CMI. Other nonatherosclerotic conditions which can also cause acute mesenteric vessel thrombosis include vasculitis, an extension of an intimal dissection flap, and infection.

NOMI accounts for 10–20% of acute bowel ischemia [31]. It is characterized by the presence of ischemia and necrosis in nonconsecutive wide areas of the bowel with no occlusion of the mesenteric artery or vein supplying the effected region. Vasoconstriction with associated decreased blood flow is felt to be the underlying condition. Conditions that predispose a patient to NOMI include sepsis, cardiac failure, hypotension, hypovolemia, and use of vasoconstrictive drugs. NOMI should be suspected in a critically ill patient with abdominal pain and/or distention and evidence of multi-organ dysfunction [30].

Mesenteric venous occlusive disease is the cause of less than 10% of AMI. Virchow's triad of venous stasis, endothelial injury, and hypercoagulability are the most common causes and can be due to a multitude of disease processes. Venous stasis may be due to portal hypertension, bowel inflammation, pancreatitis, abdominal surgery, or sepsis. Numerous medications, malignancies, and hematologic conditions render a patient hypercoagulable.

AMI can be a difficult diagnosis to make. Due to the high mortality, the suspicion must be high particularly in patients with abdominal pain out of proportion to the physical exam. A thorough history and physical exam are essential and can help in differentiating the possible pathologic process resulting in ischemic bowel. Laboratory studies should include a basic metabolic panel, complete blood count, coagulation tests, liver function tests, amylase, lipase, serum lactate, and D-dimer. These tests are not specific for AMI, however, may reaffirm suspicion or suggest an alternate diagnosis. Up to 90% of patients with AMI will have an elevated white blood cell count, and 88% will have metabolic acidosis with elevated lactate levels [32].

Contrast-enhanced computer tomography (CT) of the abdomen and pelvis is essential in the evaluation of suspected AMI and should be performed as early as possible in the clinical course. CT is a rapid exam which is widely available and has a high sensitivity (93%) and specificity (100%) for detecting and diagnosing AMI [33, 34]. Multiphasic CTA is ideal; however, a routine contrast-enhanced CT if CTA is not available will also be beneficial. Multiphasic CTA protocols will vary by institution but often include a precontrast phase, arterial phase, and delayed venous phase. The noncontrast phase is used to evaluate vascular calcifications, intramural hemorrhage, and dense thrombus. During the arterial phase, CT images are acquired when the IV contrast is most concentrated in the arterial vasculature. This allows for careful evaluation of the anatomy, detection of filling defects within the contrast pool indicative of thrombus, and preprocedural planning if necessary. The data set from the arterial images can be used to create three-dimensional reconstructions which can also be used in preprocedural planning. Delayed phase images are obtained at a predetermined time interval following IV contrast injection. This set of images will show end-organ perfusion or lack thereof, evidence of inflammation, or suggest an alternate diagnosis. Intestinal pneumatosis and portal venous gas are strong indicators of advanced AMI and can be seen on all phases of a CTA if present as can a pneumoperitoneum suggesting bowel perforation.

Contrast-enhanced CT is contraindicated in patients with a history of anaphylactic reaction to IV contrast. In this subset of patients, a noncontrast CT can be performed which may show bowel edema with or without pneumatosis intestinalis or portal venous gas. Contrast-enhanced CT/CTA should be performed on patients with chronic renal insufficiency or those on dialysis. Due to the high mortality rate of AMI, the risk of delayed or missed diagnosis outweighs the risk of contrast-induced nephropathy.

Once the diagnosis is confirmed, fluid resuscitation is initiated with crystalloids and blood products to enhance visceral perfusion and avoid cardiovascular collapse. Electrolyte and acid–base status should be assessed and corrected. Broad-spectrum antibiotics should be given immediately as the breakdown of the intestinal mucosal barrier facilitates bacterial translocation and increases the risk of sepsis [35]. Surgical intervention is first-line therapy if there is evidence of bowel necrosis and peritonitis. In patients without evidence of peritonitis, several endovascular options exist including aspiration embolectomy, thrombolysis, angioplasty, and stent placement.

Step 1. Arterial Vascular Access and Sheath Selection

A femoral, brachial, or radial approach may be chosen. Sheath size and length will depend on the size of the therapeutic device to be used and access site.

Step 2. Selection of the SMA

The SMA can be selected using a variety of diagnostic catheters including reverse curve catheters, such as the Sos Omni Selective (AngioDynamics, Latham, NY, USA), an angled glidecath (Terumo, Elkton, MD, USA), or C1 (Cook) depending on operator preference. Once selected and angiogram is performed to delineate the anatomy and location of the thrombus. A 0.035 hydrophilic guidewire is then advanced into the ileocolic branch of the SMA. If a glidecath or C1 was initially used, the catheter can be carefully advanced over the wire, and the hydrophilic wire exchanged for a more stable 0.035 wire such as a Rosen or Bentson wire. A reverse curve catheter may not easily track over the wire or may have an unfavorable angle for wire exchange. Care must be taken during exchanges to avoid dissection of the vessel which could impede blood flow to segments of bowel that were not affected by the original ischemic event (Figure 7.6).

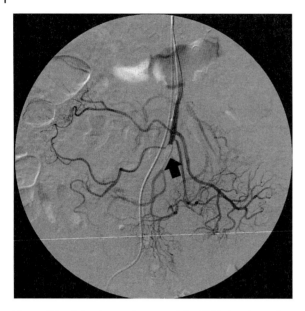

Figure 7.6 Selective angiogram of the SMA showing a thrombus (arrow) in the distal vessel.

Step 3. Aspiration Embolectomy

Several methods and devices are available for thrombus aspiration. In the absence of a dedicated thrombectomy device, a 7 Fr 45 cm sheath is advanced over the wire (if not already initially used for vascular access. A longer sheath will be necessary if brachial or radial access is used). The sheath should be carefully advanced proximal to the thrombus in the SMA. A 6 Fr guiding catheter is then advanced over the wire and into the clot. The wire is removed and a 20 cc syringe is connected to the guiding catheter. Aspiration of the guiding catheter is performed as it is withdrawn through the thrombus. The guiding catheter should be completely removed from the patient. Any clot within the catheter should be expelled, and the catheter flushed thoroughly. The flow switch on the sheath should be opened to allow back-bleeding of any retained clot. An angiogram is performed to evaluate for residual thrombus. If present, aspiration through the guide catheter can be repeated after replacing the wire (Figure 7.7).

Dedicated thrombectomy catheters such as the Export (Medtronic, Minneapolis, MN, USA) and 5MAX ACE (Penumbra, Alameda, CA, USA) have also been used with success. The Export catheter has a dual lumen design which allows for the guidewire to remain in place while thrombus is aspirated through the second lumen. This design facilitates multiple passes without having to replace a wire in

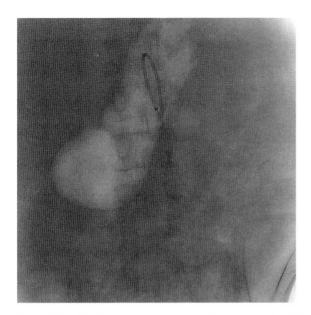

Figure 7.7 6 Fr 55 cm vascular sheath advanced into the SMA via a right femoral approach. A Penumbra thrombectomy catheter has been placed coaxially and is used to aspirate thrombus.

between aspirations. The 5MAX ACE catheter is available in several sizes with the largest inner diameter size of 0.068″. Aspiration of the Penumbra family of catheters is facilitated through a proprietary pump system. Once the Penumbra aspiration catheter is advanced to the level of the thrombus, the wire is removed, and the aspiration tubing is connected to the catheter. The pump is turned on and the thrombus is aspirated. In both aspiration systems, the device should be completely withdrawn from the patient's body. Any clot should be expelled and the catheter flushed before reintroducing it for another sweep if necessary.

Step 4. Angiogram

A postaspiration angiogram is performed. A residual disease can be treated with angioplasty, thrombolysis, or stent placement (Figures 7.8 and 7.9).

Step 5. Thrombolysis

A hydrophilic guidewire is advanced through the thrombus. A variety of multi-sidehole infusion catheters are available including standard infusion and an EKOS ultrasound augmented infusion catheter (BTG, London, UK). A treatment

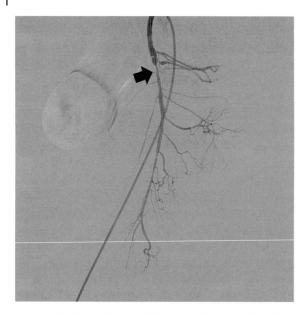

Figure 7.8   Residual stenosis (arrow) after aspiration of thrombus.

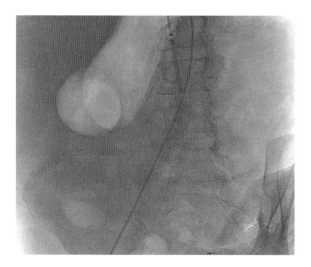

Figure 7.9   Angioplasty of stenotic lesion in SMA using Savvy 5 mm × 4 cm angioplasty balloon (Cordis, Milpitas, CA) over a V-18 wire.

length of 10 cm is sufficient. After confirming the catheter positioning, the wire can be removed, and infusion started. If an EKOS catheter is used, the wire is exchanged for a transducer wire. The transducers emit a high-frequency, low ultrasound energy which loosens the fibrin lattice within the clot. This enhances the penetration of the thrombolytic agent and exposes more plasminogen receptor sites. Recombinant tissue plasminogen activator (TPA) is the most commonly used lytic agent. TPA is infused through the catheter directly into the thrombus at a rate of 0.5–1 mg/h.

Step 6. Infusion and Follow-Up

Infusion times can range from 12 to 24 hours and can be done in a monitored unit setting. The vascular access sheath and infusion catheter should be secured to prevent accidental movement or dislodgment. The patient can then be transferred out of the angiography suite as TPA is infusing. During infusion, arterial punctures should be avoided. Fibrinogen and partial thromboplastin time (PTT) should be monitored every six hours. If fibrinogen levels fall below 150, the TPA dose should be halved, and if below 100 – TPA should be discontinued. After completing the infusion, the patient will return for an angiogram, and treatment of any underlying stenosis with angioplasty or stent placement.

Stent placement, if necessary, should be done with a balloon-expandable stent. The principles of stent placement are similar to CMI.

Mesenteric Venous Thrombosis

If a diagnosis of mesenteric venous thrombosis is made, and there is no evidence of peritonitis, medical management with anticoagulation is first-line therapy. The use of intravenous systemic intravenous TPA has been reported with success [36], though is rarely used due to risk of bleeding. If signs of peritonitis develop, emergency surgery with resection of necrotic bowel is indicated. If the patient is not improving with anticoagulation alone, a trans-jugular intrahepatic portosystemic shunt (TIPS) can be placed followed by thrombectomy and/or lysis of the mesenteric venous clot. The shunt will function as a low-resistance outflow tract for the effected mesenteric vein. The technique of TIPS placement is beyond the scope of this chapter.

Follow-Up and Outcomes

Patients will require lifelong therapy depending on the etiology of AMI. Embolic disease will necessitate anticoagulation therapy with coumadin or an alternate. Those patients with arterial thrombosis should be treated with a statin and an antiplatelet agent [28]. Patients with AMI treated with endovascular therapy have a 12.3% in-hospital mortality rate compared with 33.1% for open surgical revascularization. Endovascular therapy is also associated with a lower mean hospitalization cost and decreased risk of acute renal failure [37].

References

1 Zelenock, G.B., Graham, L.M., Whitehouse, W.M. Jr. et al. (1980). Splanchnic arteriosclerotic disease and intestinal angina. *Arch. Surg.* 115: 497–501.

2 Pillai, A.K., Kalva, S.P., Hsu, S.L. et al. (2008). Quality improvement guidelines for meseteric angioplasty and stent placement for the treatment of chronic mesenteric ischemia. *J. Vasc. Interv. Radiol.* 19: 642–647.

3 Thomas, J.H., Blake, K., Pierce, G.E. et al. (1998). The clinical course of asymptomatic mesenteric arterial stenosis. *J. Vasc. Surg.* 27: 840–844.

4 Rose, M.K., Pearce, B.J., Matthews, T.C. et al. (2015). Outcomes after celiac artery coverage during thoracic endovascular aortic aneurysm repair. *J. Vasc. Surg.* 62: 36–42.

5 Nakamura, T., Hirano, S., Noji, T. et al. (2016). Distal pancreatectomy with en bloc celiac axis resection (modified Appleby procedure) for locally advanced pancreatic body cancer: a single-center review of 80 consecutive patients. *Ann. Surg. Oncol.* 23 (suppl 5): 969–975.

6 Schermerhorn, M.L., Giles, K.A., Hamdan, A.D. et al. (2009). Mesenteric revascularization: management and outcomes in the United States, 1988–2006. *J. Vasc. Surg.* 50: 341–348.

7 Alahdab, F., Arwani, R., Pash, A.K. et al. (2008). A systemic review and meta-analysis of endovascular versus open surgical revascularization for chronic mesenteric ischemia. *J. Vasc. Surg.* 67: 1598–1605.

8 American College of Radiology. ACR Appropriateness Criteria® Radiologic management of mesenteric ischemia. https://acsearch.acr.org/docs/69501/Narrative/revised 2022.

9 Pecoraro, F., Ancic, Z., Lachat, M. et al. (2013). Chronic mesenteric ischemia: critical review and guidelines for management. *Ann. Vasc. Surg.* 27: 113–122.

10 Atkins, M.D., Kwolek, C.J., LaMuraglia, G.M. et al. (2007). Surgical revascularization versus endovascular therapy for chronic mesenteric ischemia: a comparative experience. *J. Vasc. Surg.* 45: 1162–1171.

11 Silva, J.A., White, C.J., Collins, T.J. et al. (2006). Endovascular therapy for chronic mesenteric ischemia. *J. Am. Coll. Cardiol.* 47: 944–950.

12 Aburahma, A.F., Campbell, J.E., Stone, P.A. et al. (2013). Perioperative and late clinical outcomes of percutaneous transluminal stentings of the celiac and superior mesenteric arteries over the past decade. *J. Vasc. Surg.* 57: 1052–1061.

13 Sarac, T.P., Altinel, O., Kashyap, V. et al. (2008). Endovascular treatment of stenotic and occluded visceral arteries for chronic mesenteric ischemia. *J. Vasc. Surg.* 47: 485–491.

14 Grilli, C.J., Fedele, C.R., Tair, O.M. et al. (2004). Recanalization of chronic total occlusions of the superior mesenteric artery in patients with chronic ischemia: technical and clinical outcomes. *J. Vasc. Interv. Radiol.* 25: 1515–1522.

15 Mendes, B.C., Oderich, G.S., Tallarita, T. et al. (2018). Superior mesenteric artery stenting using embolic protection device for treatment of acute or chronic mesenteric ischemia. *Society for Vascular Surgery* 678 (4): 1071–1078. https://doi.org/10.1016/j.jvs.2017.12.076.

16 Oderich, G.S., Tallarita, T., Gloviczki, P. et al. (2012). Mesenteric artery complications during angioplasty and stent placement for atherosclerotic chronic mesenteric ischemia. *J. Vasc. Surg.* 55: 1063–1071.

17 Oderich, G.S., Bower, T.C., Sullivan, T.M. et al. (2009). Open versus endovascular revascularization for chronic mesenteric ischemia: risk-stratified outcomes. *J. Vasc. Surg.* 49: 1472–1479.

18 Peck, M.A., Conrad, M.F., Kwolek, C.J. et al. (2010). Intermediate-term outcomes of endovascular treatment for symptomatic chronic mesenteric ischemia. *J. Vasc. Surg.* 51: 140–146.

19 Bieble, M., Oldenburg, W.A., Paz-Fumagalli et al. (2007). Surgical and interventional visceral revascularization for the treatment of chronic mesenteric ischemia-when to prefer which? *World J. Surg.* 31: 562–568.

20 Fioole, B., van de Rest, H.J., Meijer, J.R. et al. (2010). Percutaneous transluminal angioplasty and stenting as first-choice treatment in patients with chronic mesenteric ischemia. *J. Vasc. Surg.* 51: 386–391.

21 Sharafuddin, M.J., Olson, C.H., Sun, S. et al. (2003). Endovascular treatment of celiac and mesenteric arteries stenoses: applications and results. *J. Vasc. Surg.* 38: 692–698.

22 Matsumoto, A.H., Angle, J.F., Spinosa, D.J. et al. (2002). Percutaneous transluminal angioplasty and stenting in the treatment of chronic mesenteric ischemia: results and longterm followup. *J. Am. Coll. Surg.* 194 (1 suppl): S22–S31.

23 Oderich, G.S., Erdoes, L.S., Lesar, C. et al. (2013). Comparison of covered stents versus bare metal stents for treatment of chronic atherosclerotic mesenteric arterial disease. *J. Vasc. Surg.* 58: 1316–1323.

24 Turba, U.C., Saad, W.E., Arslan, B. et al. (2012). Chronic mesenteric ischaemia: 28-year experience of endovascular treatment. *Eur. Radiol.* 22: 1372–1384.

25 Horton, K.M. and Fishman, E.K. (2007). Multidetector CT angiography in the diagnosis of mesenteric ischemia. *Radiol. Clin. North Am.* 45: 275–288.

26 Schoots, I.G., Koffeman, G.I., Legemate, D.A. et al. (2004). Systematic review of survival after acute mesenteric ischaemia according to disease aetiology. *Br. J. Surg.* 91: 17–27.

27 Beaulieu, R.J., Arnaoutakis, K.D., Abularrage, C.J. et al. (2014). Comparison of open and endovascular treatment of acute mesenteric ischemia. *J. Vasc. Surg.* 59: 159–164.

28 Acosta, S. (2015). Mesenteric ischemia. *Curr. Opin. Crit. Care* 21: 171–178.

29 Clair, D.G. and Beach, J.M. (2016). Mesenteric Ischemia. *N. Engl. J. Med.* 374: 959–968.

30 Bala, M., Kashuk, J., Moore, E. et al. (2017). Acute mesenteric ischemia guidelines of the World Society of Emergency surgery. *World J. Emerg. Surg.* 12: 38–49.

31 Peters, J.H., Reilly, P.M., and Merine, D.S. (1991). *Textbook of Gastroenterology*. Philadelphia: Lippincott.

32 Kougias, P., Lau, D., El Sayed, H.F. et al. (2007). Determinants of morbidity and treatmet outcome following surgical interventions for acute mesenteric ischemia. *J. Vasc. Surg.* 46: 467–474.

33 Aschoff, A.J., Stuber, G., Becker, B.W. et al. (2009). Evaluation of acute mesenteric ischemia: accuracy of biphasic mesenteric multi-detector CT angiography. *Abdom. Imaging* 34: 345–357.

34 Menke, J. (2010). Diagnostic accuracy of multidetector CT in acute mesenteric ischemia: systematic review and meta-analysis. *Radiology* 256: 93–101.

35 Silvestri, L., van Saene, H.K., Zandstra, D.F. et al. (2010). Impact of selective decontamination of the digestive tract on multiple organ dysfunction syndrome: systematic review of randomized controlled trials. *Crit. Care Med.* 38: 1370–1376.

36 Hmoud, B., Singal, A.K., and Kamath, P.S. (2014). Mesenteric venous thrombosis. *J. Clin. Exp. Hepatol.* 4: 257–263.

37 Erben, Y., Protack, C.D., Jean, R.A. et al. (2018). Endovascular interventions decrease length of hospitalization and are cost-effective in acute mesenteric ischeia. *J. Vasc. Surg.* 68: 459–469.

8

Aorto-Iliac Interventions

Michael S. Segal[1], Sameh Elrabie[1], and Rajesh K. Malik[2]

[1] *Department of General Surgery, Wyckoff Heights Medical Center, Brooklyn, NY, USA*
[2] *Division of Vascular Surgery, Wyckoff Heights Medical Center, Brooklyn, NY, USA*

Introduction

Obtaining computed tomographic angiography (CTA) improves preprocedural planning for aortoiliac disease. Planning should include anticipating any potential pitfalls and including potential bailout options in the plan. Access should be obtained dependent on the lesion location determined from preprocedural imaging and may require multiple sites of access. Shorter, less complex lesions are best treated with a self-expandable stent. Longer, complex, calcified lesions are better treated with covered stents and protect against potential rupture during deployment. If you require precise deployment, then consider using a balloon-expandable stent.

Preoperative Workup

Preprocedural planning and imaging is key to performing successful aortoiliac interventions. This workup begins with diagnostic studies to assess the disease location, extent of disease, calcifications, and gain an appreciation for potential pitfalls that may be encountered during therapeutic intervention [1]. Appropriate preprocedural workup can reduce contrast load for the patient, radiation exposure to the provider, and improve safety and success rates.

Endovascular Interventions: A Step-by-Step Approach, First Edition. Edited by Jose M. Wiley, Cristina Sanina, George D. Dangas, and Prakash Krishnan.
© 2023 John Wiley & Sons Ltd. Published 2023 by John Wiley & Sons Ltd.

Noninvasive Studies

Computed Tomographic Angiography

Computed tomographic angiography (CTA) has become the most utilized imaging modality for preoperative planning. A CTA provides substantial information, including potential access-related issues, length and complexity of the lesion, extent of calcifications, and the size of the vessels. This essential information can help minimize procedure-related complications by helping formulate a safe strategy to treat. We strongly recommend obtaining CTA imaging prior to interventions (Figure 8.1).

> **Key Point:** Obtaining a high-quality CTA allows for thorough preoperative planning.

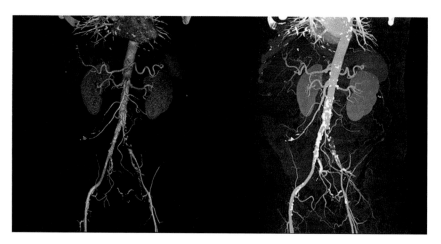

Figure 8.1 A 3D reconstruction of CTA imaging demonstrating extensive calcifications and an occluded left iliac artery.

Ultrasound Duplex

Ultrasound (US) is another imaging modality that can be used in the initial part of the workup, however, from a practical standpoint, is limited in its utility for aortoiliac interventions. This is secondary to being user dependent and limited by patient habitus above the inguinal ligament. Additionally, bowel gas patterns can limit the utility of US. An exercise ankle-brachial index may be more helpful if there is suspicion of a proximal lesion.

Magnetic Resonance Angiography

Magnetic resonance angiography is not routinely used in our practice as there is no benefit over CTA, which is easier to obtain and, in our view, provides much more useful information.

Invasive Imaging

Angiography

Angiography is rarely used in planning unless a CTA or MRA was not able to be performed. During angiography, morphologic characteristics of the diseased segments and pressure gradients can be measured to assess questionable iliac lesions. A pressure gradient of 20 mmHg or greater is considered significant [2]. In our practice, aortoiliac angiogram is performed with the intention to treat, unless the disease encountered is not amenable to endovascular intervention.

Classification of Lesion and Planning of Intervention

TransAtlantic InterSociety Consensus II Classification (TASC II)

TASC A and B lesions were amenable to endovascular interventions with positive outcomes and patency rates. Historically, TASC C and D lesions were treated with open surgical intervention. As endovascular interventions have improved, increasingly complex lesions are being approached endovascularly. TASC C and D lesions can now be treated endovascularly with patency rates approaching surgical patency rates [3] (Figure 8.2).

Planning for the Intervention

After the imaging has been reviewed, a treatment plan should be formulated. This plan should include the location of the access and the basic equipment that needs to be used during the procedure, including wires, balloons, and various stents. It is important to have appropriate bailout equipment available should a complication be encountered. This includes having larger sheaths available, covered stents, and an aortic occlusion balloon.

Step 1. Patient Factors

Aortoiliac interventions are best performed with light sedation. This is important because significant pain during the intervention, such as ballooning the artery, may indicate that the artery is stretching beyond its threshold and could risk rupture.

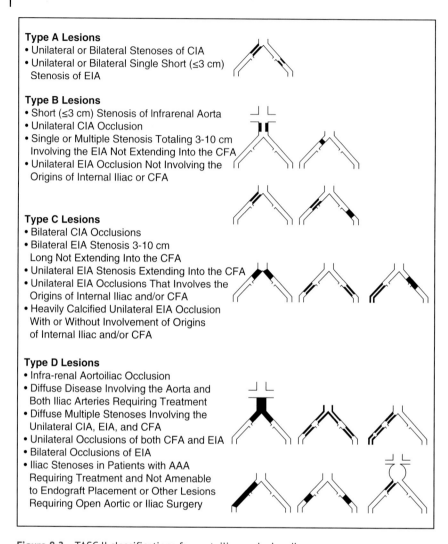

Type A Lesions
- Unilateral or Bilateral Stenoses of CIA
- Unilateral or Bilateral Single Short (≤3 cm) Stenosis of EIA

Type B Lesions
- Short (≤3 cm) Stenosis of Infrarenal Aorta
- Unilateral CIA Occlusion
- Single or Multiple Stenosis Totaling 3-10 cm Involving the EIA Not Extending Into the CFA
- Unilateral EIA Occlusion Not Involving the Origins of Internal Iliac or CFA

Type C Lesions
- Bilateral CIA Occlusions
- Bilateral EIA Stenosis 3-10 cm Long Not Extending Into the CFA
- Unilateral EIA Stenosis Extending Into the CFA
- Unilateral EIA Occlusions That Involves the Origins of Internal Iliac and/or CFA
- Heavily Calcified Unilateral EIA Occlusion With or Without Involvement of Origins of Internal Iliac and/or CFA

Type D Lesions
- Infra-renal Aortoiliac Occlusion
- Diffuse Disease Involving the Aorta and Both Iliac Arteries Requiring Treatment
- Diffuse Multiple Stenoses Involving the Unilateral CIA, EIA, and CFA
- Unilateral Occlusions of both CFA and EIA
- Bilateral Occlusions of EIA
- Iliac Stenoses in Patients with AAA Requiring Treatment and Not Amenable to Endograft Placement or Other Lesions Requiring Open Aortic or Iliac Surgery

Figure 8.2 TASC II classifications for aortoiliac occlusive disease.

Step 2. Vascular Access

In planning aortoiliac interventions, access site selection is an important consideration. Options for access include femoral, brachial, or radial arteries. Radial access is an up-and-coming option but still slightly limited by equipment lengths, although that is changing rapidly. Terumo® makes a 6 Fr 119 cm R2P Destination slender sheath® with a 5 Fr outer diameter. Through this a self-expandable stent, up to 8 mm, can be deployed to the iliac arteries. In our practice, we typically use either femoral or brachial artery access, occasionally requiring multiple access sites. The location of the lesion and anatomic factors will ultimately determine which access site is preferable [2].

Access site selection is determined by the location of the lesion. A common iliac lesion is treated from the ipsilateral common femoral artery (CFA) or brachial artery. An external iliac lesion is treated from the contralateral CFA or brachial artery. If the lesion is in the proximal portion of the external iliac artery, an ipsilateral approach can be considered. Multiple access sites may be necessary when treating more complex lesions extending up to and including the infrarenal aorta. In these cases, bilateral femoral artery access or a combined brachial and femoral access can be utilized.

There are considerations for access to reduce complications. Access is performed under US guidance. When performing brachial access and utilizing a larger sheath, 6 Fr or greater, particularly in women, we recommend a cutdown to minimize complications. That seems to be the cutoff size based on our personal experience.

Sheath selection through which the intervention is done is an important consideration for the procedure. For ipsilateral interventions of the common iliac artery, a 7 Fr radio-opaque Brite-Tip® sheath is our ideal selection. The Brite-Tip sheath or another marker tipped sheath aids in visualization of the sheath tip so that a stent is not inadvertently deployed within the sheath. This sheath is large enough to facilitate the balloon and stent sizes for the iliac artery, including the larger covered stents that are utilized as bailout options if needed. A 23 cm sheath length works well as it can be used to cross the lesion and facilitate delivery of a balloon-mounted stent without the stent dismounting off the balloon. If access from the contralateral groin is needed for an up and over approach, a 6 or 7 Fr long sheath will suffice.

> **Key Point:** Utilize appropriate access dependent on lesion location and use a sheath size to accommodate potential bailout options.

Step 3. Crossing the Lesion

Once access is obtained a suitable wire is used to cross the lesion. The wire can be supported with a catheter providing additional support and directional control. We prefer to use a 0.038/0.035-in. platform in our practice; however, smaller 0.018- or 0.014-in. wires can also be utilized in certain situations. After the lesion has successfully been crossed, a stiff 0.035-in. wire should be used to support interventions. This helps allow the devices to track across the lesion and provides a platform for rapid upsizing of a sheath should a complication be encountered.

There are additional devices that can aid in crossing of a difficult lesion. When dealing with an occlusion, one may enter a subintimal plane and at times re-entry into the true lumen can be complex. There are adjunctive devices that can assist in re-entry in these difficult circumstances. The Cordis Outback Re-entry catheter® and Phillips Pioneer Plus Intravascular Ultrasound (IVUS) Re-entry catheter® are two such devices that aid in re-entry. The Pioneer Plus has the added benefit of utilizing IVUS to visualize and direct re-entry [4]. If re-entering at the level of the aorta, we try to keep the entry point as close to the aortic bifurcation as possible to prevent creating a large dissection which could potentially propagate and become problematic.

Once the lesion is crossed, the sheath should be upsized to facilitate delivery of treatment devices. At this point the patient should be anticoagulated; in our practice, we typically heparinize the patient as this agent is easily reversible should any complication arise. We typically use 70 units/kg or less to heparinize the patients since the procedure should be relatively quick once the lesion is crossed.

Prior to treatment a complete diagnostic angiogram of the lower extremity must be performed to differentiate posttreatment emboli from preexisting lesions.

Step 4. Intervention

An initial treatment plan should be formulated prior to intervention based on preoperative imaging. Once the lesion has been crossed and an angiogram is performed, the final treatment plan is either confirmed or altered depending on extent and complexity of the lesion. Based on the quality of the preoperative imaging, rarely is the plan dramatically altered.

The typical vessel diameter for the common iliac arteries ranges from 7 to 12 mm. The arteries typically taper down to the CFA with a vessel diameter of 4–9 mm.

The options for treatment are balloon angioplasty, self-expanding (SE) bare-metal stents, SE covered stents, balloon-expandable (BE) noncovered stents, and BE covered stents (Figure 8.3). Balloon angioplasty alone is rarely used as a final modality given the superior results with stents [5]. There is less embolization, less risk of rupture, reduced overall complication, and higher long-term patency when stenting. There is some experience with primary treatment of balloon angioplasty with Shockwave® and drug-coated balloon angioplasty, but not enough to justify recommendation over stenting.

There are at present two landmark trials that have created the precedence for the selection of stents utilized for iliac stenting.

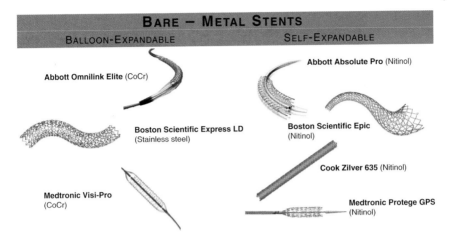

Figure 8.3 Commonly used bare-metal stents.

The *Journal of Vascular Surgery* in 2016 published the Covered vs Balloon Expandable Stent Trial (COBEST). The study concluded that patients who were treated with covered stents had a lower rate of restenosis followed out to five years [6]. The difference became even more profound as the complexity of the lesion increased. TASC C and D lesions saw the greatest benefit from a covered stent (Figure 8.4) versus bare-metal stent.

The Iliac, Common, and External Artery Stent Trial, commonly referred to as the ICE Trial, published in 2017 compared SE versus BE stents. The study found that at 12 months there was a statistically significant difference in the rate of

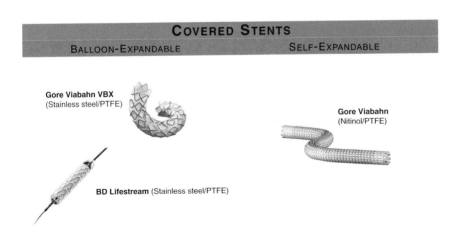

Figure 8.4 Commonly used covered stents for iliac intervention.

restenosis, 6.1% for SE stents and 14.9% for BE stents [7]. However, in heavily calcified lesions, there may not be much benefit for SE stents.

As a result of these studies, classification of the lesion being treated is important in determining what type of stent will be selected. For more shorter, less complex, and minimally calcified lesions, the utilization of a self-expandable stent provides improved patency rates. For longer, more complex, and heavily calcified lesions, the utilization of a covered stent provides a more durable treatment and protects against risk of rupture. In general, in the common iliac artery, when we require precise placement at the ostium or to avoid covering the internal iliac artery, we prefer to use BE stents. In the external iliac artery, we prefer to use SE stents, and if heavily calcified, we use a covered SE stent which is more amenable to bending at the level of the groin.

Other considerations involve the use of specialized devices to aid in the treatment of specific pathologies. One such device is Shockwave angioplasty. This device allows for balloon angioplasty with lithotripsy delivered to a calcified vessel wall. This can be used in vessel preparation prior to stent deployment by improving vessel compliance [8]. An additional treatment option, however off IFU, that can be considered is the use of an Endologix AFX Unibody Endograft® for TASC D lesions. There were promising results with primary patency rates of greater than 90% at one year [9].

The kissing iliac stents is being used with less frequency; however, the indication and utility should be recognized on a case-by-case basis. If there is disease involving the aortic bifurcation or proximal common iliac arteries, then the use of kissing iliac stents may be necessary to avoid compromising the contralateral side [10]. One must consider the need for endovascular peripheral arterial interventions in the future, as kissing iliac stents raising the bifurcation can limit the ability to go up and over in the future, but with advancement in radial access equipment this may become a moot point.

> **Key Point:** Shorter, less complex lesions are best treated with a self-expandable stent. Longer, complex, calcified lesions are better treated with covered stents and protect against potential rupture during deployment. If precise deployment is required, consider utilizing a BE stent.

Step 5. Closure

There are numerous percutaneous closure devices available. Depending on access sheath size and the quality of the vessel, calcifications, or plaque, a passive or active closure device can be utilized.

Step 6. Complications

When performing endovascular interventions there are potential complications that should be accounted for and planned for prior to the intervention. This is a list of potential complications and the management options if encountered.

Rupture

When dealing with a chronic total occlusion (CTO) or heavily calcified lesion in the aortoiliac system, the risk of rupture carries higher morbidity compared to interventions below the inguinal ligament. This should be planned for in advance by having appropriate bailout options available which can reduce the risk of a catastrophic outcome. Preoperative imaging should provide baseline characteristics about the lesion. Selection of a sheath size that can accommodate a covered stent should the lesion rupture during angioplasty is a critical bailout consideration. In our practice, when we are ballooning and have concern for rupture, we deflate, keeping the balloon in place and perform an angiogram through the sheath. If extravasation is seen, the same balloon can be quickly inflated allowing for more time until a bailout plan is initiated. If the rupture is significant you may need to get an aortic occlusion balloon which is supported by an appropriate size long sheath from a contralateral access. A long sheath helps to support the balloon so that it remains at the location you inflated it and doesn't slip down with the aortic pressure. This may give you some time to get control of the bleeding with a large, covered stent from the ipsilateral side. Monitoring the patients' blood pressure throughout the case should be done routinely. Any hypotension during the intervention of the aortic-iliac system could be indicative of a potential rupture.

Embolization

Prior to any intervention, an angiogram of the runoff down to the level of the foot should take place establishing a baseline. This prevents any postintervention confusion trying to determine if there was a preexisting lesion versus an acute embolization. If there is an embolization then endovascular techniques should be employed to salvage it.

Access Complications

Management of access-related complications extends beyond the scope of this overview. To help minimize the risk of access-related complications, percutaneous access should be performed under US guidance. Most small sheath access complications can also be managed endovascularly or conservatively and rarely require surgical intervention.

Cases

Case 1

This is a 66-year-old male with a past medical history of diabetes and long-standing smoking history. Patient had a right lower wound. Evaluation of his critical limb ischemia began with an ankle-brachial index (ABI) and arterial duplex. Arterial duplex demonstrated severe stenosis of the right external iliac artery. A CTA was unable to be obtained secondary to the patient having an acute kidney injury and elevated creatinine levels. The decision was made to undergo conventional angiogram.

Access was obtained using US guidance in the left CFA. A 5 Fr sheath inserted. An aortogram was obtained demonstrating an occlusion of the entire right external iliac artery (Figure 8.5). A complete lower extremity angiogram was performed. We were unable to cross the lesion from antegrade access, so an ipsilateral access of the right CFA was obtained, slightly lower than normal. Working from above and below the lesion was crossed. The right groin sheath was exchanged for a 6 Fr sheath with a marker tip. Initial treatment was with balloon angioplasty of the right external iliac artery and followed with a 10 mm SE stent. A completion angiogram demonstrated a good result and completion runoff angiogram was performed (Figures 8.5 and 8.6).

Case 2

This is a 57-year-old male who had presented with lifestyle limiting claudication with thigh and buttock pain. Patient was unable to ambulate more than one-half

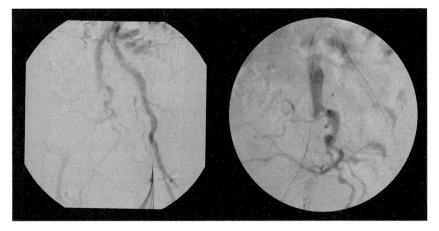

Figure 8.5 Aortogram with right external iliac artery occlusion. Through and through access obtained.

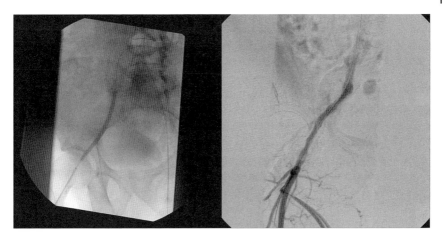

Figure 8.6 Balloon angioplasty of lesion and completion angiogram following placement of 8 mm bare-metal stent.

of a block before interfering with his job. On examination the patient had a nonpalpable left femoral pulse. ABIs were reduced on left lower extremity. A CTA was obtained (Figure 8.7). This demonstrated a greater than 50% stenosis of the right common iliac artery and occluded left common iliac artery.

Access was gained to bilateral CFA under US and fluoroscopic guidance. Five Fr sheaths were inserted and a glidewire and catheter were used to cross the right iliac artery stenosis. A diagnostic angiogram was obtained and then the left occluded iliac artery was crossed using an 0.035-in. glidewire. We then exchanged

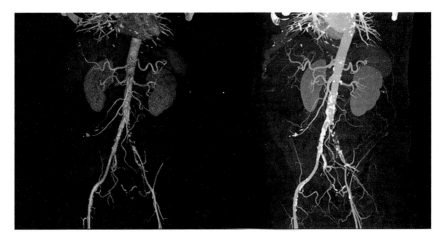

Figure 8.7 Preoperative CTA with reconstruction demonstrating occluded left common iliac artery and stenosis of the right common iliac artery.

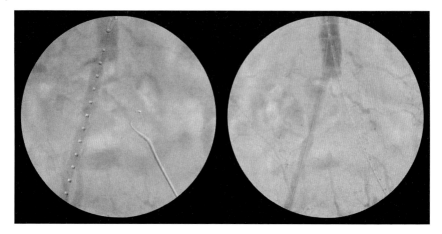

Figure 8.8 Aortogram with occluded left iliac artery and imaging with Amplatz wire in place with marker pigtail for measurement.

out for Amplatz® wires bilaterally. A marker pigtail catheter was used to obtain an accurate measurement for our stents (Figure 8.8).

We then upsized to 8 Fr sheaths bilaterally. The patient was then systemically heparinized. After confirming the length of the lesions, we advanced two 11 m × 79 mm VBX stents® in the bilateral common iliac arteries. We then retracted our sheaths. We obtained a diagnostic angiogram to confirm the location of the hypogastric arteries bilaterally. The stents were simultaneously deployed (Figure 8.9). The left hypogastric artery was occluded and correlated with preoperative imaging. A completion

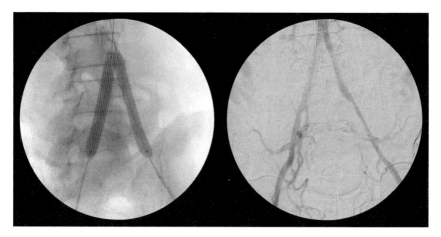

Figure 8.9 Deployment of bilateral VBX stents and completion angiogram with patent iliac arteries.

angiogram was performed and the arteriotomies were closed with Perclose® closure devices. We decided to use VBX stents since we needed precise deployment at the aortic bifurcation and the complex calcified lesion on the left side.

References

1 Gerhard-Herman, M.D., Gornik, H.L., Barrett, C. et al. (2017). 2016 AHA/ACC guideline on the management of patients with lower extremity peripheral artery disease: executive summary: a report of the American college of cardiology/American heart association task force on clinical practice guidelines. *J. Am. Coll. Cardiol.* 69 (11): 1465–1508.

2 Sidawy, A.N. and Perler, B.A. (2018). *Rutherford's Vascular Surgery and Endovascular Therapy*, 9e. Elsevier.

3 Leville, C.D., Kashyap, V.S., Clair, D.G. et al. (2006). Endovascular management of iliac artery occlusions: extending treatment to TransAtlantic Inter-Society Consensus class C and D patients. *J. Vasc. Surg.* 43 (1): 32–39.

4 Jacobs, D.L., Motaganahalli, R.L., Cox, D.E. et al. (2006). True lumen re-entry devices facilitate subintimal angioplasty and stenting of total chronic occlusions: initial report. *J. Vasc. Surg.* 43 (6): 1291–1296.

5 Deloose, K., Bosiers, M., Callaert, J. et al. (2017). Primary stenting is nowadays the gold standard treatment for TASC II A & B iliac lesions: the definitive MISAGO 1-year results. *J. Cardiovasc. Surg. (Torino)* 58 (3): 416–421.

6 Mwipatayi, B.P., Sharma, S., Daneshmand, A. et al. (2016). Durability of the balloon-expandable covered versus bare-metal stents in the Covered versus Balloon Expandable Stent Trial (COBEST) for the treatment of aortoiliac occlusive disease. *J. Vasc. Surg.* 64 (1): 83–94.e1.

7 Krankenberg, H., Zeller, T., Ingwersen, M. et al. (2017). Self-expanding versus balloon-expandable stents for iliac artery occlusive disease: the randomized ICE trial. *JACC Cardiovasc. Interv.* 10 (16): 1694–1704.

8 Brodmann, M., Werner, M., Brinton, T.J. et al. (2017). Safety and performance of lithoplasty for treatment of calcified peripheral artery lesions. *J. Am. Coll. Cardiol.* 70 (7): 908–910.

9 Maldonado, T.S., Westin, G.G., Jazaeri, O. et al. (2016). Treatment of aortoiliac occlusive disease with the Endologix AFX unibody endograft. *Eur. J. Vasc. Endovasc. Surg.* 52 (1): 64–74.

10 Haulon, S., Mounier-Véhier, C., Gaxotte, V. et al. (2002). Percutaneous reconstruction of the aortoiliac bifurcation with the "kissing stents" technique: long-term follow-up in 106 patients. *J. Endovasc. Ther.* 9 (3): 363–368.

9

Femoropopliteal Arterial Interventions in the Claudicant

Sahil A. Parikh, Joseph J. Ingrassia, and Matthew T. Finn

Division of Cardiovascular Diseases, Columbia University Irving Medical Center, New York, NY, USA

Introduction

Endovascular intervention has become the preferred initial therapy for the invasive treatment of femoropopliteal disease, with bypass surgery commonly reserved for complex or refractory lesions [1]. Patients with peripheral arterial disease are now 4× more likely to receive endovascular approach rather than an open surgical treatment of their disease [2]. This clinical demand has driven device development creating numerous treatment options available for the proceduralist [3]. Despite significant technologic improvements, the femoropopliteal vascular segment presents unique biomechanical challenges for lasting definitive treatment given the complex forces on the vessel from the adjacent joint movements [4, 5]. In this chapter, we describe in detail the indications, approaches, imaging technologies, and devices which may be used to approach pathology in the femoropopliteal vessel. Furthermore, we entail the available evidence surrounding their use.

Patient Evaluation and Indications for Treatment of Femoropopliteal Arterial Pathology

The patient evaluation centers on the standard history and physical evaluation. Classical historical symptoms of femoropopliteal obstructive disease involve exertional symptoms in the calf and foot. Claudication may be described as a burning or cramping discomfort brought on by exertion and improved with rest. In more severe cases, symptoms may be aggravated by elevation and improved with dependent positioning. Symptomatology may be atypical in a significant percentage of patients, particularly those with comorbidities affecting pain receptor function (i.e. spinal stenosis and diabetic neuropathy). The patient exam will demonstrate diminished pulses below the affected area typically in the popliteal and pedal segments. Temperature in the affected limb may be reduced and the limb may develop distal pallor when elevated. The skin may also lose dermal appendages appearing hairless and dry with brittle discolored nails on the affected feet. An ankle brachial index may be performed bedside or in the vascular laboratory by taking the ratio of the higher upper extremity Dopplered systolic pressure over the higher of the Dopplered systolic pressures between the dorsalis pedis and the posterior tibial artery. Finally, the neurologic assessment of sensory and motor function is an essential component of a comprehensive vascular exam.

Classical vascular imaging involves vascular ultrasound with Doppler assessment. Computed tomography with lower extremity runoff can also be helpful for precise imaging of the lower extremities and is particularly useful for the aortoiliac and femoropopliteal segments.

Indications for Revascularization
Femoropopliteal Claudication

The 2016 American Heart Association/American College of Cardiology guidelines for the treatment of peripheral arterial disease provide a IIa recommendation for revascularization of claudication for patients with an inadequate response to goal-directed medical treatment defined as supervised exercise program, aspirin, cilostazol (in those without a contraindication), and intensive comorbidity management (diabetes, hyperlipidemia, blood pressure management, as well as smoking cessation) [6].

The recently released multi-societal appropriate use criteria for peripheral intervention [1] grant an "M" designation for "May Be Appropriate" to the superficial femoral artery (SFA) and popliteal arterial chronic total occluded segments for endovascular or surgical treatment of symptoms despite goal-directed medical therapy. In nonoccluded femoropopliteal segment lesions, endovascular treatment is escalated to "A" for "Appropriate" for symptoms despite goal-directed medical treatment.

Vascular Imaging in Endovascular Treatment

Contrast Angiography

Fluoroscopic angiography with use of contrast remains the first-line tool for the endovascular operator. Digital subtraction imaging (DSA) is utilized and enhances vascular visualization by subtracting the bony or dense structures from the image [7].

DSA can also reduce the amount of dye required for image acquisition. Even with less contrast delivered, full-strength contrast injections into the extremity tend to be painful. A 50/50 mix of contrast and saline with DSA can allow for diagnostic images while reducing patient discomfort.

CO_2 Angiography

Peripheral arterial disease is prevalent in the chronic kidney disease populations [8, 9]. CO_2 angiography presents an attractive alternative to enable successful peripheral arterial disease intervention without the need for contrast dye exposure. Furthermore, CO_2 can be useful in patients with severe contrast allergies [10].

CO_2 angiography has important limitations. First, it may require specialized software to visualize the CO_2. Second, medical grade CO_2 cannot be delivered via mechanical power injection; and therefore, manual injection must be performed to achieve imaging. Third, in order to prevent erroneous air injection into the arterial system, one must create a separate system of tubing and syringes to allow for purging of atmospheric air and the creation of a closed CO_2-filled circuit. Importantly, caution should be observed if a patient complains of abdominal pain after a CO_2 injection, as this could be a sign of intestinal ischemia related to successive injections of CO_2 [11]. Therefore, one should generally have a delay of two to three minutes between subsequent CO_2 injections [12]. Finally, imaging of the infratibial vessels is generally limited with CO_2 and may require switching the system to contrast or utilizing direct injection of CO_2 with a catheter placed in the below-the-knee popliteal artery [13].

Steps to CO_2 Angiography

1) Switch system imaging setting for CO_2 detection.
2) Set up separate tubing for introduction and purging of CO_2. The CO_2 cartridges can be contained in a sterile bag on the procedure table (Figure 9.1a) with the sterile tubing attached.
3) One may use two large tubes and a one-way valve at the end of the tubing, usually comes with the set to purge the system of air and fill it with CO_2; Figure 9.1b.
4) Perform DSA angiography using hand injections from the syringe (Figure 9.1c).

Extravascular and Intravascular Ultrasound

Extravascular ultrasound (EVUS) has become a critical tool in safe arterial access and efficient vascular access [14]. Intraprocedural use of EVUS can also be useful in achieving procedural success by allowing controlled intraluminal wire reentry for complex chronic total occlusion crossing [15].

(a)

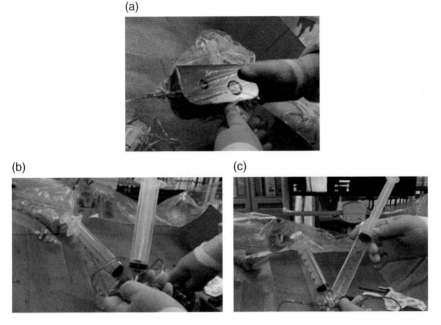

(b)   (c)

Figure 9.1 CO_2 angiography (a) The device is placed in a sterile bag on the working table with the CO_2 cartridge attached. (b) Connect two large syringes to a three-way stopcock for filling the system completely with CO_2. A one-way valve sits on the end of the catheter for connection to the catheter in the body. (c) Fill one of the syringes with CO_2 and purge the system of atmospheric air. Hand inject the CO_2 with the large syringe while capturing the image.

Intravascular ultrasound (IVUS) is a valuable tool in endovascular assessment of accurate vessel sizing, stenosis area determination, and visualization of the composition of arterial plaque (Figure 9.2). Preintervention IVUS precisely determines vessel size. This may be particularly important for self-expanding stents with less radial force than balloon-expandable scaffolds and can avoid both under- and over-sizing [16–18]. IVUS may also inform atherectomy, angioplasty, or lithotripsy device selection by evaluating the degree of calcification within a stenotic segment.

Steps to IVUS Use

Three IVUS sizes are available: standard 0.014″ IVUS, which is also useful in the coronaries, is produced by multiple companies. There are 0.018″ and 0.035″ IVUS systems available from both Boston Scientific and Phillips. The 0.035″ IVUS is useful for large vessels and veins and is typically not necessary for the femoro-popliteal segment.

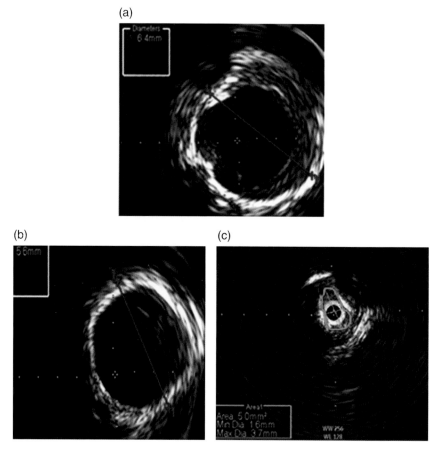

Figure 9.2 Example of the measurements typically taken with intravascular imaging on preintervention assessment. (a) Proximal reference diameter assessment (b) Distal reference diameter assessment (c) pre-procedural minimal lumen area assessment.

1) Ensure adequate anticoagulation and administer vasodilators prior to use, typically 100–200 mcg nitroglycerin intraarterially (as long as no contraindication exists).
2) Place the IVUS catheter beyond the lesion. Prior to entering the body perform adequate catheter flushing and ensure functionality.
3) Manual pullback is generally performed given the length of imaging runs required in the femoropopliteal segments. Radiolucent measuring tape placed on the leg is used to coregister the IVUS with the angiogram. Bookmarks can be captured every 100 mm during pullback to correspond with marking tape measurements.

4) After pullback is completed, one may reintroduce the IVUS and fluoro-store the catheter tip location to determine the exact location of the vessel ostia (if pertinent to the case) or lesion segments. This technique can be useful in reducing contrast in patients with chronic renal insufficiency.

5) Next remove the catheter from the body and bleed back from the sheath to prevent introduction of air.

6) Measurements can then be performed and include the distal reference diameter, proximal reference diameter, and minimal lumen area (Figure 9.2a–c). There is currently insufficient data to recommend exactly how reference measurements should be taken based on lumen measurement or based on external elastic lamina.

7) One may also utilize IVUS images to assess severity, arc, and length of calcification. This may aid in decision-making regarding pretreatment with atherectomy or the potential need for specialty/lithotripsy balloons [19].

8) After treatment, repeat IVUS passes are used to assess for dissection, posttreatment minimal lumen, or stent diameters [20].

Vascular Access and Lesion Crossing Techniques

A variety of vascular access options and crossing techniques exist to enable success despite challenging anatomy. This section will describe the various access for crossing lesions and their steps.

Steps for Crossover "Up and Over" technique

The "Up and Over" Crossover technique for peripheral intervention is the most common and traditional form of access and method of crossing.

1) Obtain common femoral access contralateral to the symptomatic side or lesion of interest based on noninvasive testing. Place a short sheath typically 4–6 Fr using modified Seldinger technique over the access wire.

2) Perform ipsilateral runoff if needed. One can place the image intensifier at 30° ipsilateral to the access site to open the bifurcation of the SFA and profunda arteries.

3) Next perform an inflow aortogram. Place an Omni Flush catheter (Angiodynamics, Latham, NY, USA), ImagerII catheters (Boston Scientific), or a pigtail at the T12 or L1 vertebrae. Have the patient perform an expiratory breath hold. DSA imaging is performed with the injection of about 20 cc of 50/50 contrast/saline for visualization. Keys to an ideal diagnostic aortogram are high field of view, vertical orientation of the image intensifier, raised table

to decreased magnification by increasing the signal to object distance. The tip of the catheter should be positioned at the top of the screen so that the full field of view is used.

4) After the contralateral iliac is wired, bring down the catheter to the top of the femoral head and move the image intensifier to 30° ipsilateral of the vascular segment of interest. Often a contralateral shot should also be taken for further delineation of the anatomic segment of interest. If the decision is made to intervene, advance a soft tipped, stiff wire through the catheter into a safe distal vessel in the contralateral leg. For proximal SFA stenosis, one may place the wire carefully in the profunda to allow for adequate wire "purchase." Next place a long-braided sheath "up and over" to the desired segments. For proximal SFA interventions a 40–50 cm sheath is used. For more distal interventions, longer sheaths may be chosen to enhance pushability when crossing high-grade stenoses.

Radial

The radial approach for endovascular interventions is an excellent alternative to femoral access. Unfavorable iliac tortuosity may be overcome more easily from the radial approach. Challenges to radial access remain especially in terms of available equipment, including adequate device length, compatible drug-coated devices, and embolic protection filters [21].

Steps for Radial Approach:

1) Left radial access is preferred for these cases as it does not require traversal of the aortic arch thereby minimizing distance to the abdominal aorta. Ultrasound imaging may be useful to confirm the radial arterial diameter is at least 25 mm to accommodate long specialty sheaths commonly utilized for these procedures.
2) Once radial access is obtained place a radial specific short sheath into the proximal vessel.
3) Use a JR4 or similar shaped catheter to traverse the subclavian artery and engage the descending aorta with a 0.035″ wire.
4) Advance an exchange length wire followed by a catheter to the descending aorta.
5) Abdominal aortography may be performed with a long pigtail catheter or a sidehole multipurpose catheter (ensure the tip is free from small branches before performing large injections).
6) Complete bilateral diagnostic runoff angiography to assess for disease by cannulating bilateral iliacs with a long sidehole catheter.
7) Use a stiff 0.035″ guidewire (e.g. Supra Core [Abbott, Chicago, IL, USA], glidewire advantage [Terumo, Shibuya City, Japan], or a long stiff glidewire [Terumo])

to advance the radial intervention sheath (typically 119 or 149 cm R2P destination sheath, Terumo) proximal to the femoropopliteal segment of interest.

8) Once the sheath is positioned, various strategies can be deployed to cross the diseased vascular segment.

Tibio-Pedal Approach

The tibio-pedal approach for distal entry to a stenosis or occlusion is a necessary component for more complex peripheral intervention. Given the retrograde cap of chronic total occlusions is typically softer than the proximal cap, utilizing pedal access can significantly add to crossiblity of complex and long segment chronic occlusions.

Steps to retrograde access and wire crossing (Figure 9.3).

1) Ultrasound the tibial vessels to determine if retrograde access is feasible and the best vessel to initially attempt. Study of preintervention ultrasound is critical in determining vessel approach and runoff patency. In general, in patients with single vessel runoff, one may try to avoid tibio-pedal access and sheath placement, as injury to this vessel could lead to acute limb ischemia.

2) If all three below-the-knee vessels are patent, one may access in the anterior tibial preferentially at or above the ankle joint for easiest closure after the procedure is complete (Figure 9.3a–c). Local anesthesia is given to anesthetize the access arterial segment (Figure 9.3c). The posterior tibial artery is our second choice followed by peroneal. The peroneal artery is typically done under fluoroscopic guidance by puncturing directly between the tibia and fibula distally.

3) After access using ultrasound guidance, one can wire under fluoroscopy and place a tibial access sheath. A radial access sheath (Figure 9.3e–f) may also be repurposed for pedal access. Give a vasodilator cocktail (i.e. 200 mcg of nitroglycerin, assuming no contraindication) and perform angiography distally through the pedal sheath.

4) Next utilize a 0.014″ or 0.018″ wire coupled with a crossing catheter to gain access to the distal cap of an occlusion or stenosis to facilitate distal crossing.

Antegrade Femoral Access

Antegrade femoral arterial access allows for ipsilateral intervention sparing the need for crossing-over technique. Antegrade sheath location can enhance support to allow advancement of equipment and may be particularly useful for popliteal and below-the-knee occlusive disease.

Antegrade access may be obtained with ultrasound guidance with the probe in a transverse position allowing visualization of the femoral head, common

(a)   (b)   (c)

(d)   (e)   (f)

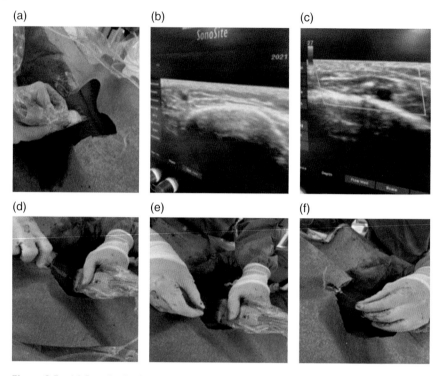

Figure 9.3 (a) Prep in the foot and ultrasound. (b, c) Visualization of the anterior tibial artery (d) Local anesthesia directed to the access vessel. (e–f) Needle access to the vessel can be obtained using axial or longitudinal ultrasound views. Axial imaging and access is demonstrated here.

femoral, and superficial femoral/profunda bifurcation. This will ensure safe entry in a compressible segment of the vessel and enable steering into the SFA [22]. Standard short sheaths can be utilized. Access into the common femoral rather than the superficial femoral access may help avoid vascular access complications such as pseudoaneurysms if closure devices are not utilized, however, may require more radiation and longer access times as the access wire tends to move toward the profunda [23].

Working Wire Size and Changing Between Systems

An important consideration in peripheral interventions is size of the working wire utilized after lesion crossing. In coronary artery interventions, 0.014″ is the standard wire size. In peripheral intervention, operators use crossing catheters to change between wire sizes for compatibility of specialty balloons and atherectomy equipment. See Tables 9.1 and 9.2 for a list of wire sizes associated with various commonly used devices.

Lesion Preparation

Plain Old Balloon Angioplasty

Attempting to reduce vascular dissection with plain old balloon angioplasty (POBA) is important, given registry data demonstrating that up to 40% of patients may require bailout stenting due to dissections after POBA [24, 25]. In general,

Table 9.1 Examples of wire sizes and device types.

Device	0.014″	0.018″	0.035″
Semi-compliant peripheral balloons[a]	Yes	Yes	Yes
Dorado			Yes
Drug-coated balloons[a]		Yes	Yes
Angiosculpt balloon	Yes	Yes	
Wolverine	Yes		
Vascutrak	Yes	Yes	
Ultrascore	Yes		Yes
Chocolate	Yes	Yes	
Shockwave	Yes		
SpiderFx filter	Yes (specialty spider wire replaces 0.014)		
Emboshield	Yes (specialized Bare Wire or 0.014″ with 0.018″ tip viper wire)		
Peripheral IVUS (Boston Scientific)	Yes	Yes	Yes
Peripheral IVUS (Philips)	Yes	Yes	Yes
Bare-metal stents[a]	Yes	Yes	Yes
Supera		Yes	
Eluvia DES			Yes
Zilver DES			Yes
Tack			Yes
Covered stents[a]	Yes	Yes	Yes

[a] Size varies based on individual specifications by manufacturer. Note: list is not comprehensive. Device manufacturers: Dorado, Vascultrack, and Ultrascore (B-D), Angiosculpt (Philips), Wolverine, Chocolate, SpiderFx (Medtronic), Emboshield and Supera (Abbott), Eluvia (Boston Scientific), Zilver (Cook).

Table 9.2 Major plaque modification/atherectomy devices, specifications, and utilization for peripheral arterial disease.

Device	Mechanism	Rail guidewire size (inches)	Sheath size	Eccentric calcium	CTO lesion with subintimal segment	Thrombotic lesions efficacy	ISR lesions	BTK lesions
Excimer laser	Monochromatic light to dissolve/soften plaque	0.014″	6 Fr	Yes	Yes	Yes	Yes	Yes
Rotablator	Rotational	Specialty wire: tapered wire with 0.014″ spring tip	Depends on burr size. 6 Fr sheath generally acceptable					Yes
JetStream	Rotational	0.014″	7 Fr	Yes		Yes	Yes	
Phoenix	Rotational	Specialty wire: 0.014″	5–7 Fr depending on device size				Yes	
Rotarex	Rotational	Specialty wire, 0.018	6 Fr or 8 Fr depending on device			Yes		
Ocelot	Rotational – OCT image guide	0.014″	6 Fr	Yes	Yes			
Pantheris	Directional – OCT image guided	0.014″	7 or 8 Fr	Yes	Yes			

HawkOne	Directional	0.014″	7 fr LS, LX 6 fr M, S	Yes	Yes (face toward true lumen)
Diamondback 360	Orbital	0.014″ with 0.018″ tip	4 Fr 1.25 mm burrs 5 Fr 1.25, 1.75 mm burrs and all radial compatible burrs 6 Fr 2.0 mm burr	Yes	Yes

Abbreviations: CTO – chronic total occlusions; ISR – in-stent restenosis, BTK – below-the-knee, Fr – French, OCT – optical coherence tomography.
Source: Adapted with permission Finn et al. Interv Cardiol Clin. 2020 Apr;9 [2]:125–137 Excimer Laser and Phoenix (Philips), Rotablator and Jetstream (Boston Scientific), Rotarex (B-D), Ocelot/Pantharis (Avinger), HawkOne (Medtronic), Diamondback360 (Cardiovascular Systems, Inc).

POBA is optimally performed at lower pressures with longer inflation times minimizing the number of balloon inflations. This "doctrine" of optimal POBA is based on several small studies showing less vascular dissection with these techniques. Longer versus shorter inflation times were evaluated in a study of less than versus greater than three minutes [26]. Significant dissections occurred less often (22.7% vs. 50.9%, p < 0.001) in the long inflation group [26]. The effect of balloon length on vascular dissections was also evaluated in a study of de novo femoropopliteal stenosis based on the theory that fewer balloon inflations would lead to less dissection at the edge of the treatment segments. One study showed that long balloons (≥220 mm) requiring fewer serial inflations had a significantly decreased incidence of severe dissection than with short balloons (<150 mm) and multiple inflations (47.1% vs. 70.0%, p = 0.019) [27].

Focal Force Balloons for Optimal Lumen Gain

Focal balloons such as cutting, scoring, and lithotripsy balloons are often used in the treatment of femoropopliteal diseased segments. These technologies are utilized to treat refractory lesions and may prevent dissections by avoiding "watermelon seeding" (balloon slipping) which may occur with semi-complaint peripheral balloon inflation [28].

Data for use of these technologies is primarily registry based, single arm, and nonrandomized; however, despite these limitations, these devices show promising results. One study of scoring balloons had an 82.1% one-year patency in patients with femoropopliteal disease (Figure 9.4a) [29]. The chocolate balloon (Medtronic – Minneapolis, MN, USA, Figure 9.4b), a semi-compliant balloon within a nitinol cage, was evaluated in the Chocolate BAR registry [30] and demonstrated a 93.1% freedom from stenting postangioplasty. High-pressure noncompliant balloons such as the Dorado Kevlar balloon (Figure 9.4c, B-D, Franklin Lakes, NJ, USA) may also be useful in treatment of refractory stenoses and may be more deliverable due to the lack of metal caging present on scoring balloons.

The ShockWave lithotripsy balloon (Figure 9.4d, ShockWave Medical, Santa Clara, CA, USA) was examined in the DISRUPT PAD III registry which was recently presented. The study showed statistical superiority of intravascular lithotripsy when compared to POBA on the primary endpoint of procedural success in severely calcified vascular segments. The study also reported significantly improved post-ballooning diameter, arterial dissection, and less bailout stenting than POBA [31].

Drug-Coated Balloons

Drug-coated balloons (DCBs) have been shown to be superior in numerous studies when compared to POBA. A meta-analysis demonstrated clear efficacy of DCB in decreased late lumen loss and rates of target vessel revascularization [32]. Recently,

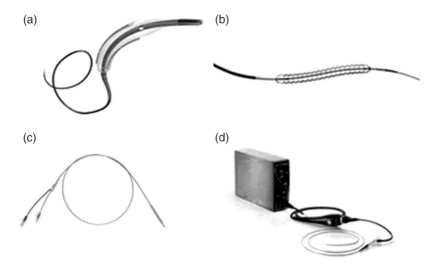

Figure 9.4 (a) Cutting balloon example (b) Chocolate balloon (c) Dorado high-pressure noncompliant Kevlar balloon (d) Shockwave intravascular lithotripsy. *Source:* Reproduced with permission from Medtronic, Inc., (c) B-D, (d). Reproduced with permission from ShockWave Medical Inc.

paclitaxel-coated balloons received a black box warning following a meta-analysis with a signal of higher mortality in comparison to POBA [33]. Several pooled analysis and meta-analyses have refuted these results. Furthermore, a recent large, multicenter randomized controlled trial showed no difference in mortality between paclitaxel-coated balloons compared to mortality in over 2289 randomized patients [34]. The US Food and Drug Administration (FDA) recently approved an additional DCB for market release, signifying regulatory confidence in these devices.

Atherectomy

Endovascular plaque modification and atherectomy utilizes a variety of mechanisms to debulk, soften, crack, remove, vaporize, or otherwise modify the vessel structure in order to improve device passage and increase luminal gain with angioplasty balloons or stents [35]. These benefits may come with higher associated risk, i.e. vessel perforation or distal embolization. Currently available marketed device types for atherectomy include: laser, directional, rotational, and orbital atherectomies.

Laser
Laser-guided PM (Excimer, Philips, Amsterdam, Netherlands, Figure 9.5a) utilizes pulses of monochromatic light to "vaporize" vascular plaque or tissue. Laser was the first extensively studied "atherectomy" device in the field.

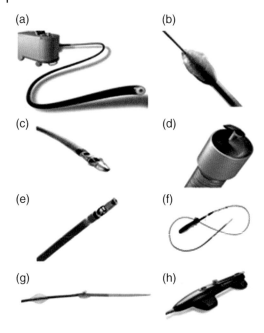

Figure 9.5 (a) Excimer laser, (b) Rotablator (c) Jetstream (d) Phoenix (e) Rotarex (f) HawkOne (g) Pantheris (h) Diamondback360. *Source:* Images compliments of their respective device companies (see text). Adapted from Finn et al. (2020), with permission from Elsevier.

The single-arm CELLO study [36] enrolled 65 patients with moderate-to-severely calcified femoropopliteal disease. The study demonstrated a primary patency rate of 76.9% at one year. The EXCITE study [37] randomized 250 patients with femoropopliteal in-stent restenosis (ISR) to excimer laser plus POBA versus POBA alone. Freedom from target lesion revascularization (TLR) at six months was: 73.5% versus 51.8% favoring laser + POBA ($p = 0.05$). This trial importantly demonstrated superiority of laser atherectomy for treatment of ISR and supported this additional FDA indication.

Excimer Laser Use Steps

1) After crossing lesions, swap out for 0.014″ or 0.018″ wire and place an embolic protection device if needed (embolic protection typically requires specialty wires depending on the device used, see below).
2) Provide protective glasses to staff. Ensure all involved have undergone appropriate laser safety training. The laser should remain in standby or off mode when not in use so not accidentally activated outside of the body.

3) Catheter options include turbo-power and turbo-elite catheters which are 7 Fr and 6 Fr, respectively. The turbo-power catheter has an additional hand control to allow the laser head to pivot.

4) Next, connect a saline syringe to the flush port. One should have several 10 ml syringes ready for longer runs.

5) Calibrate the device outside of the body. Wear protective glasses throughout the procedure and look away from the beam during calibration.

6) Place the catheter in the body, activate the laser with the foot pedal and then apply slow forward pressure advancing the device through the lesion at a rate of about 1–2 mm/s. While advancing, one should gently flush the saline port. Whenever active atherectomy is being used fluoroscopy imaging should be performed.

7) After passing through the lesion, angiography may be done to assess for complications and to determine if repeat passes are required.

Rotational Atherectomy

Several rotational atherectomy systems are marketed in the United States. The rotablator system (Figure 9.5b) is available for use in infrainguinal (particularly below-the-knee) disease. A classic French study of 150 patients reported a high complication rate (25%) with rotational atherectomy; however, complications were very broadly defined [38].

JetStream atherectomy (Boston Scientific, Marlborough, MA, USA, Figure 9.5c) uses rotational atherectomy combined with active aspiration of released debris. The device has been examined in two registries: JET and JET-SCE [39, 40]. In JET, 241 patients with de novo or restenotic lesions received treatment and one year primary vessel patency was 77.2% based on duplex ultrasound. JET-SCE enrolled patients receiving Jetstream plus DCB versus Jetstream atherectomy plus POBA. The 12-month incidence of TLR free survival was 94.7% for Jetstream + DCB versus 68.0% for Jetstream plus POBA (p = 0.002).

The Phoenix system (Philips, Amsterdam, Netherlands, Figure 9.5d) also combines front-end lesion cutting with debris clearance. This device was studied in the 2014 EASE registry [41] which demonstrated an 88% six-month freedom from TLR and had a low-rate embolization (<1%). A recent retrospective study examined rotational atherectomy + DCB versus DCB alone in 226 patients with femoropopliteal disease undergoing treatment with the Phoenix atherectomy device. The studies showed higher technical success rates and lower rates of bailout stenting in the atherectomy plus DCB arm compared to DCB alone (technical success 95.4% vs. 84.8%, p = 0.006; bailout stenting 5.1% vs. 20.6%, p < 0.001) [42].

The Rotarex device (B-D, Franklin Lakes, NY, USA, Figure 9.5e) was recently approved in the United States and has a long track record in Europe. Like Jetstream and Phoenix, the device combines rotational atherectomy cutting with plaque and thrombus removal. It was recently studied in combination with DCBs in a small group of patients with chronic total occlusions and ISR. After one year, the restenosis rate determined by duplex ultrasonography was 20.5% with 5.5% rate of TLR.

Rotational Atherectomy Steps

1) Select appropriate sheath size and wire for the desired device. Place embolic protection distal to the lesion if desired.
2) Test the device outside of the body off the drape or towels to ensure functionality. Jetstream, Rotarex, and Phoenix have additional tubing for active aspiration functions of the device.
3) Rotablator burr may be chosen based on vessel size. Burrs are available in 1.25, 1.5, 1.75, 2.0, 2.15, 2.25, 2.38, and 2.5 mm sizes. Because the burr should be sized approximately to 2/3rds the size of the vessel diameter. Even the largest burrs may not be large enough for the femoropopliteal segments which have somewhat limited the use of the device above-the-knee. Of note, the 2.38 and 2.50 burrs are recommended for 8 Fr sheaths and the 2.00–2.25 mm burr fit through 7 Fr.
4) Pass the device through the lesion according to device specifications. Rotablator requires a rapid engagement and disengagement "pecking motion" of lesions. With rotablator, avoid decelerations which may be associated with distal embolization or device entrapment.
5) The Jetstream has a "blades-up" feature which can be utilized after an initial successful "blades-down" pass to increase luminal gain.

Directional Atherectomy

The HawkOne Directional atherectomy line of devices (Medtronic, Minneapolis, MN, USA, Figure 9.5f, Diamondback360 orbital atherectomy Figure 9.5h) and Pantheris (Avinger, Redwood City, CA, USA, Figure 9.5g) are examples of directional atherectomy devices which use rotating cutting disks to resect and then remove the atherosclerotic plaque. The HawkOne utilizes one-directional cutting blade consisting of a rotating blade inside a housing with a collection area. An activating switch starts the cutting and when engaged allows the device to "jog" toward the wall and engage plaque for removal by the device. The HawkOne comes in several sizes and lengths depending on the segment designated for treatment [43].

In the single-arm DEFINITIVE-LE study, 797 patients with claudication or critical limb ischemia (CLI) underwent Hawk directional atherectomy [44]. At one year, primary patency rate was 78% among claudicants and 71% in patients with CLI. The subsequent DEFINITIVE-AR [45] multicenter randomized controlled pilot trial compared directional atherectomy + DCB versus DCB alone in 102 patients with calcified femoropopliteal lesions. The study showed no difference between treatment arms but was underpowered. DEFINITIVE-AR did, however, find that directional atherectomy plus DCB had a significantly lower incidence of flow limiting dissection compared to DCB alone (p = 0.01). The incidence of procedural embolization requiring treatment in the atherectomy arm was extremely rare (n = 2), although distal embolic protection filters were deployed to prevent this in more than 80% cases.

The Avinger (Redwood City, CA, USA) Pantheris directional atherectomy system utilizes optical coherence tomography with directional atherectomy. The imaging component is designed to allow for targeted atherectomy of diseased vessel segments. The Pantheris device was studied in the 2017 VISION trial. This study showed a 97% procedural success rate with only a 4% rate of TLR at six months, although lesions with moderate to severe calcification were excluded [46].

Steps to directional atherectomy with HawkOne system:

1) Choose the correct sheath size based on the size of device desired. 7 Fr for HawkOne Ls and Lx; 6 Fr for HawkOne M and S (note L denotes "Large," M denotes "Medium," S denotes "Small," Lx denotes "Large Long," and Ls denotes "Large short" for the collection chamber/device working area. The Lx can be used in long lesions so the device can perform more atherectomy without filling the collection chamber).

2) The Hawk systems can be used over any 0.014″ wire; however, the device is frequently used in conjunction with 0.014″ embolic protection specialty wires.

3) One can consider performing IVUS to identify the location and composition of the lesion prior to Hawk atherectomy.

4) Flush the device and prior to placement on the wire ensure the tip of the nose cone is aligned with the collection chamber.

5) First, pass the device through the lesion in the off position to ensure it will pass easily and not get stuck. If it will not pass, one may try an undersized balloon inflation in the index lesion to aid in passage. When inflating the balloon, first go to low pressure and examine where the balloon is compressed by the stenosis. This will serve as an additional hint as to where directional atherectomy should be focused.

6) Once the device is able to pass through the stenotic segment in the off position, position the device with the cutting portion just proximal to the lesion. The lesion may be turned 360° using the dial just proximal to the hand controller. Be careful to not overturn the dial, which can cause wire wrap and prevent easy advancement of the device.

7) To initiate the atherectomy turn on the hand controller at the base and pull-back on the orange "On" switch. Be sure to give adequate back tension on the orange switch to engage the device by activating the "jog" toward the lesion.

Cutting should only be performed in the proximal to distal direction. Multiple passes or "cuts" can subsequently be performed facing different portions of the vessel wall. Care should be taken to avoid large branches or aneurysmal segments as this may lead to arterial perforation. Of note, if unable to engage the lesion adequately, ensure the access sheath is back far enough proximally to allow the "jog" of the device to fully engage the lesion.

8) A radiolucent marker on the collection chamber moves back toward the device handle as the chamber fills with plaque. Once the collection chamber is nearly full, remove the device and position the flush port over the distal catheter. Open the flush port by un-aligning the nose tip from the collection port and flush hard to remove the debris. The device can then be reintroduced for additional passes if needed.

9) Angiography should be performed periodically to evaluate treatment effectiveness, to rule out perforation and distal embolization.

10) After directional atherectomy, ballooning or stenting may be used if necessary for definitive treatment.

Orbital Atherectomy

The Diamondback360 orbital atherectomy (Cardiovascular Systems Inc., St. Paul, MN, USA, Figure 9.5h) device orbits in a 360° arc inside the vessel. The Diamondback360 atherectomy is marketed in multiple crown sizes, shapes, and lengths for different lesion subsets. The device is also available in long shaft length to allow for treatment of the lower extremity from the radial artery.

Compliance360 was a small randomized pilot study of patients with calcified femoropopliteal disease comparing Diamondback360 orbital atherectomy plus POBA versus POBA alone [47]. At six months, freedom from TLR or restenosis was achieved in 77.1% of OA group and 11.5% of POBA group ($p < 0.001$). These differences were no longer significant at one year (81.2% vs. 78.3%, $p > 0.99$). Nevertheless, investigators demonstrated that orbital atherectomy resulted in a significantly lower rate of bailout stenting (5.3% vs. 77.8%, $p < 0.001$).

Orbital atherectomy steps:

1) Using an exchange catheter, place the viper atherectomy wire. One can consider utilizing the 300 cm wire with the 0.018″ tip coupled with the Nav 6, 4–7 mm emboshield filter deployed in the P2 or P3 segment of the popliteal artery. If employing a radial approach, use the 400 cm viper wire and choose the 180 or 200 cm shaft Diamondback device.

2) The CSI comes in several different burr sizes and crowns which can be utilized for different vessels. Recently, exchangeable crowns have been released allowing the operator to treat multiple segments with different size burrs without needing to exchange for an entirely new device.

3) Next, prime the device with a proprietary lubricant solution (ViperSlide®) and, with the rear break up, walk it into the proximal aspect of the lesion. If one encounters difficulty advancing the device to the lesion, one may engage glide assist by holding down the low speed until the light button blinks, then push the black start button activating glide assist. Once in position, push the start button and again press the low-speed knob to turn off glide assist. Engage the brake.

4) One should always initially pass the lesion at a low-speed setting. Twist to release the green starting knob and tap the start button while on fluoroscopy. Pass the device slowly through the lesion at 1–3 mm/s. Unlike rotablator, slow forward progress through the lesion is preferred with the Diamondback device. The pitch of the device will change with ablation of calcified segments and therefore one may focus more ablation time on these segments.

5) Additionally, the construction of the crown allows for bidirectional cutting. The operator may pass the crown through the lesion slowly, and then, under the same run return it to the starting position.

6) Next change speeds by tapping the speed settings on the back of the device and complete additional runs as desired.

7) To treat additional vessel segments, open the brake and advance the device over the wire. Reengage the brake and begin the treating again as required.

Embolic Protection

Embolic protection is an important consideration when treating thrombotic lesions or performing atherectomy. Embolic protection is more commonly deployed when infratibial runoff is limited to one or two vessels and an atherectomy strategy is planned from the proximal to distal direction. Current technology does not allow for embolic protection use with radial or retrograde (pedal) approaches.

Several available devices are currently available in the United States; however, only two are approved for use in the lower extremity: The SpiderFx™ filter (Medtronic, MN, USA), the Emboshield NAV6™ (Abbott, MN, USA). The Wiron Device™ (Cardiovascular Systems, Inc, AK, USA) is also planned for market release and will provide an additional option for embolic protection.

Steps for use Spider Filter Fx (Medtronic, Video 9.2).

1) After crossing the lesion, swap for a 0.014″ or 0.018″ wire (can be long or short in length as the delivery system is monorail).

2) Choose the correct size filter for the vessel of interest. In the SFA popliteal, 5–7 mm filters are commonly utilized.

3) Flush the device carefully to prevent introduction of air within the filter.

4) Place the green port on the end of the 0.014″ wire while bending the catheter and ensure the wire exits at the small slit in the white stripe just distal to the green portion of the delivery catheter.

5) Insert the device as a monorail while pinning the wire. Advance the system under fluoroscopy until the black radiolucent distal end of the device is in position. Remove the 0.014″ wire and advance the spider wire carefully. Unsheath the filter and walk out the introduction catheter saving it for removal (will use the blue end). The wire has a dock that can allow the spider wire to be shortened. In peripheral procedures, it is often preferable to keep the full length of the device for over-the-wire peripheral devices.

6) Next perform your intervention/atherectomy.

7) If wire access needs to be maintained after the filter is removed, take a new workhorse wire next to the device with care not to wire into the basket (which could dislodge captured particulate and lead to distal embolization).

8) Next take the blue retrieval catheter and advance into the body, partially collapsing the filter for removal. Remove the retrieval catheter, the filter, and spider wire together.

9) Actively aspirate and bleed back the sheath to ensure no retained particulate is present.

10) Take completion angiography to evaluate for distal embolization or damage to the vessel from the filter during retrieval.

Steps for use Emboshield NAV 6 (Abbott):

1) Open the device and pour saline into the plastic surrounding the filter to flush it. Next open the syringe provided in the kit with the green funnel and flush into the filter to remove air (Figure 9.6a). Illustrated directions for flushing are provided on the sterile plastic packaging.

2) Tighten the green torquer device on the bare wire and use the wire to pull the filter collapsing it into the black delivery catheter.

3) One may then remove the short 190 cm bare wire, which comes with the filter and replace it with a long 315 cm wire (which comes separately). Of note, the bare wire contains a larger radiolucent tip than the working portion of the wire to prevent the filter from coming off the distal portion of the wire.

4) Place the 315 cm bare wire into the body through a 0.018″ or 0.035″ crossing catheter and remove the catheter. Next, advance the filter deployment catheter using monorail technique.

5) As long as the treatment zone does not include the P2 or P3 segment popliteal artery, one may deploy the filter in the space behind the knee joint where it is more easily visualized due to separation in the bone from the cartilage (Figure 9.6b).

6) To deploy the filter, position the distal back dot in the target area. Remove the red safety mechanism and pull the end of the white lever to expand the filter.

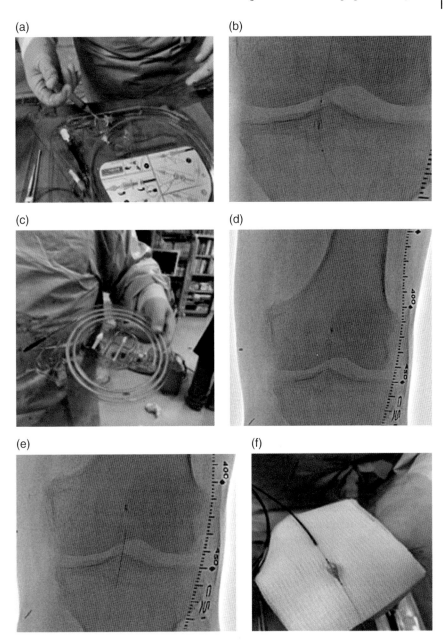

Figure 9.6 Example of Nav6 Emboshield Filter Deployment and removal. (a) Carefully flush and de-air the filter according to specifications on the device packaging. (b) Using monorail technique, deliver the filter. Pull the red safety tab off when the filter is in position and then pull on the white tab to release the filter on the wire. (c) Retrieval catheter. (d) Positioning of the retrieval catheter at the proximal radiolucent dot of the filter. (e) Pull the wire to partially collapse the filter and remove the filter with the wire under fluoroscopic visualization. (f) Push the filter out of the catheter outside the body and examine for clot or plaque.

7) Walk out the delivery catheter with care not to pull out or kink the bare wire.
8) Removing the filter (Figure 9.6c–e**)**. After treatment, the wire and the filter are typically removed together. First, advance the retrieval catheter on the wire using monorail technique. Next, place the retrieval catheter over the proximal radiolucent dot on the wire and pull the wire back slowly. The bare wire has a larger radiolucent wire tip which will pull the filter into the retrieval catheter. Leave about half of the filter outside of the catheter so as to not push out captured contents inside the filter.
9) Pull the wire, filter, and retrieval catheter out of the body together. This is typically done under fluoroscopy to ensure the filter does not get caught in vessel or stent structures during removal (Figure 9.6f).
10) Actively aspirate and bleed the sheath to ensure no retained particulate is present.

Troubleshooting Embolic Protection Devices

Two issues commonly arise with filter placement. First, the filter can become "full," preventing flow to the lower leg. Second, distal embolization can occur if the filter is accidentally advanced down a tibial artery, if the filter is undersized for the vessel, or if particulate is lost during device removal.

Troubleshooting a "Full" Filter
1) Place a second wire, near but not into the filter. On the second wire bring down an angled crossing catheter without sideholes (one can also utilize aspiration catheters for this purpose), i.e. Pneumbra (Pneumbra, San Francisco, CA, USA)), Pronto (Teleflex, Wayne, PA, USA), Export (Medtronic, Minneapolis, MN, USA), QuickCat (Philips, San Diego, CA, USA), and Fetch2 (Boston Scientific, Marlborough, MA, USA).
2) Position the tip of the angled crossing catheter just inside the filter.
3) Actively aspirate from the crossing catheter.
4) Next, one may bring the retrieval catheter and remove the filter while performing active aspiration from the angled catheter to prevent distal particulate from becoming dislodged during filter removal (see steps above).

Distal Embolization or "No Reflow"
Distal embolization can be a serious complication of femoropopliteal procedures. It can usually be managed by following several approaches. Surgical consultation for distal bypass or open embolectomy may be considered if flow is unable to be restored in a timely fashion.

1) First, if no contraindication exists one should typically give vasodilators directly into the distal vascular bed. In cases of microemboli, vasodilators alone may significantly improve flow. Generally, direct acting vasodilators such as nitroprusside or calcium channel blockers may be more effective than nitroglycerine.

2) If flow is not restored, then carefully compare the postintervention angiogram to preprocedure runoff to determine where embolization may have occurred.

3) Next, wire the selected tibial vessel(s) and consider gentle ballooning with an undersized balloon. If this is ineffective or larger scale embolization is suspected, one may utilize aspiration catheters. The Penumbra CatRx or Cat 3 over-the-wire device provides an option for aspiration thrombectomy.

4) If steps 1–3 are ineffective, one could consider obtaining retrograde pedal access and placing a sheath to give direct vasodilators beyond the lesion and for additional aspiration.

5) One can also consider alternative differentials to embolization if flow is still not restored such as dissection. IVUS may be helpful in this determination.

Stenting for Femoropopliteal Disease

Bare-Metal Stents

Current endovascular practice generally favors avoiding stent placement as first-line treatment if possible. However, important indications for stenting remain such as residual stenosis/recoil after POBA and significant dissection.

The first major study comparing vascular stenting with bare-metal stents (BMSs) to POBA alone demonstrated a markedly higher 12-month patency with BMSs compared to POBA (63% vs. 37%, p = 0.001). The RESILIENT randomized trial compared BMS with the Lifestent (B-D, Franklin Lakes, NJ, USA) to POBA. The study again showed improved primary patency at three years (75.5% vs. 41.1%, p < 0.001). The subsequent SUPERB registry examined the Supera nitinol woven stent, reported primary patency of 86.3% with zero stent fractures at one year.

Deployment of the Supera stent requires careful attention to the stent deployment with stent elongation associated with worse outcomes compared to stent compression or nominal deployment due to hypothesized loss of radial forces with elongation [48–50].

Drug-Eluting Stents (DES)

The Zilver paclitaxel drug-eluting stent (DES) (Cook Medical, Bloomington, IN, USA) was compared to optimal POBA with the option for bailout BMS. Zilver demonstrated superior patency at five years (66.4% vs. 43.4%, p < 0.001) compared to controls. This study was followed by the IMPERIAL study which compared the second-generation Eluvia DES (Boston Scientific, Marlborough, MA, USA) to Zilver. Eluvia met prespecified noninferiority criteria at one year with a primary patency of 88.5% vs. 79.5%, p for noninferiority <0.01.

Alternative Stent Technologies

Covered Stents

Covered stents are offered by several companies and come in both balloon-expandable and self-expandable versions. These can be useful in treating vascular access complications in the femoropopliteal segments with care not to exclude major vascular branches. A retrospective cohort study of stent-graft use with the Viabahn® (Gore, Newark, DE, USA) self-expanding covered stent in the above-the-knee superficial femoral and P1 popliteal demonstrated a one year patency of 81.7% [51].

Tacks

The Tack® endovascular stent (InTack Vascular, Wayne, PA, USA) is a nitinol implant 6 mm in length utilized to reappose dissection flaps. These devices were evaluated in the recently published single-arm TOBA II study, which evaluated 213 patients who received treatments with the Tacks after POBA. The study showed a one year 79.3% primary patency rate with 92.1% of lesions having complete resolution of the vascular dissection [23]. The TOBA III single-arm multi-center registry examining the Tacks in long lesions paired with subsequent treatment with DCB was demonstrated a 95.0% primary patency at a year with only one bailout stent event in the entire study.

Final Efficacy Assessment

After completing definitive treatment with POBA, focal force balloons, DCBs, or stents, the final assessment is performed with diagnostic imaging. Angiography or CO_2 imaging after definitive treatment is used to assess for residual stenosis, vascular or stent edge dissection, branch occlusion, absence of vascular perforation/hematoma, and adequate distal vessel runoff without severe embolization. IVUS can be useful to evaluate stent expansion and wall apposition as well as to understand the severity of vascular dissections after treatment. Pullback gradients or fractional flow reserve measurements may be performed before and after treatment to demonstrate adequate treatment of vascular stenoses. Finally, physical pulse assessment and extremity exam must be routinely performed and documented prior to patient transfer to the recovery area.

Conclusions

Femoropopliteal obstructive arterial disease can lead to debilitating symptoms. When optimal medical therapy is inadequate or CLI is present, endovascular treatment should be considered. The rise in popularity of endovascular procedures has caused an explosion in endovascular devices allowing a high rate of successful and durable treatment of these lesions.

Sorting through the vast catalog of options has become challenging. This chapter provides a practical reference for understanding the indications, steps for use, and data associated with common techniques in the treatment of obstructive femoro-popliteal disease.

Acknowledgments

The device companies mentioned for assistance with specification data and images.

References

1 Bailey, S.R., Beckman, J.A., Dao, T.D. et al. (2019). ACC/AHA/SCAI/SIR/SVM 2018 appropriate use criteria for peripheral artery intervention. *J. Am. Coll. Cardiol.* 73: 214–237. http://dx.doi.org/10.1016/j.jacc.2018.10.002.

2 Guez, D., Hansberry, D.R., Gonsalves, C.F. et al. (2020). Recent trends in endovascular and surgical treatment of peripheral arterial disease in the medicare population. *J. Vasc. Surg.* 71: 2178. http://dx.doi.org/10.1016/j.jvs.2020.03.015.

3 Mohan, S., Flahive, J.M., Arous, E.J. et al. (2018). Peripheral atherectomy practice patterns in the United States from the vascular quality initiative. *J. Vasc. Surg.* 68: 1806–1816. http://dx.doi.org/10.1016/j.jvs.2018.03.417.

4 Müller-Hülsbeck, S., Schäfer, P.J., Charalambous, N. et al. (2010). Comparison of second-generation stents for application in the superficial femoral artery: an in vitro evaluation focusing on stent design. *J. Endovasc. Therap.* 17: 767–776. http://dx.doi.org/10.1583/10-3069.1.

5 MacTaggart, J.N., Phillips, N.Y., Lomneth, C.S. et al. (2014). Three-dimensional bending, torsion and axial compression of the femoropopliteal artery during limb flexion. *J. Biomech.* 47 (10): 2249–2256.

6 Gerhard-Herman, M.D., Gornik, H.L., Barrett, C. et al. (2016). AHA/ACC guideline on the management of patients with lower extremity peripheral artery disease: executive summary. *J. Am. Coll. Cardiol.* 2017. 69: 1465–1508. http://dx.doi.org/10.1016/j.jacc.2016.11.008.

7 Gates, J. and Hartnell, G.G. (2000). Optimized diagnostic angiography in high-risk patients with severe peripheral vascular disease. *Radiographics* 20 (1): 121–133.

8 O'Hare, A.M., Glidden, D.V., Fox, C.S., and Hsu, C.-Y. (2004). High prevalence of peripheral arterial disease in persons with renal insufficiency: results from the national health and nutrition examination survey 1999-2000. *Circulation* 109 (3): 320–323.

9 Fowkes, F.G.R., Rudan, D., Rudan, I. et al. (2013). Comparison of global estimates of prevalence and risk factors for peripheral artery disease in 2000 and 2010: a systematic review and analysis. *Lancet* 382 (9901): 1329–1340.

10 Fujihara, M., Kawasaki, D., Shintani, Y. et al. (2015). Endovascular therapy by CO_2 angiography to prevent contrast-induced nephropathy in patients with chronic kidney disease: a prospective multicenter trial of CO_2 angiography registry. *Catheter. Cardiovasc. Interv.* 85: 870–877. http://dx.doi.org/10.1002/ccd.25722.

11 Mizuno, A., Nishi, Y., and Niwa, K. (2014). Total bowel ischemia after carbon dioxide angiography in a patient with inferior mesenteric artery occlusion. *Cardiovasc. Interv. Ther.* 29 (3): 243–246.

12 Prasad, A. (2015). CO_2 angiography for peripheral arterial imaging: the good, bad, and ugly. *Catheter. Cardiovasc. Interv.* 85 (5): 878–879.

13 Back, M.R., Caridi, J.G., Hawkins, I.F., and Seeger, J.M. (1998). Angiography with carbon dioxide (CO_2). *Surg. Clin. North Am.* 78: 575–591. http://dx.doi.org/10.1016/s0039-6109(05)70335-2.

14 Nguyen, P., Makris, A., Hennessy, A. et al. (2019). Standard versus ultrasound-guided radial and femoral access in coronary angiography and intervention (SURF): a randomized controlled trial. *EuroIntervention* 15 (6): e522–e530.

15 Mustapha, J.A., Diaz-Sandoval, L.J., and Saab, F. (2015). Extravascular Ultrasound Guidance for CTO Crossing. https://evtoday.com/pdfs/et0515_F4_Diaz.pdf (accessed 03 January 2023).

16 Garcia, L., Jaff, M.R., Metzger, C. et al. (2015). Wire-interwoven nitinol stent outcome in the superficial femoral and proximal popliteal arteries: twelve-month results of the SUPERB trial. *Circ. Cardiovasc. Interv.* 8 (5): http://dx.doi.org/10.1161/CIRCINTERVENTIONS.113.000937.

17 Indes, J. and Gates, L. (2013). New treatment of iliac artery disease: focus on the Absolute Pro® vascular self-expanding stent system. *Med. Devices Evid. Res.* 147. http://dx.doi.org/10.2147/mder.s31696.

18 Supera device speficiations. https://www.accessdata.fda.gov/cdrh_docs/pdf12/P120020c.pdf (accessed 03 January 2023).

19 Fujino, A., Mintz, G.S., Matsumura, M. et al. (2018). A new optical coherence tomography-based calcium scoring system to predict stent underexpansion. *EuroIntervention* 13 (18): e2182–e2189.

20 Shammas, N.W., Torey, J.T., Shammas, W.J. et al. (2018). Intravascular ultrasound assessment and correlation with angiographic findings demonstrating femoropopliteal arterial dissections post atherectomy: results from the iDissection study. *J. Invasive Cardiol.* 30 (7): 240–244.

21 Sher, A., Posham, R., Vouyouka, A. et al. (2020). Safety and feasibility of transradial infrainguinal peripheral arterial disease interventions. *J. Vasc. Surg.* 72 (4): 1237–46.e1.

22 Hwang, J.H., Park, S.W., Kwon, Y.W. et al. (2020). Ultrasonography-guided antegrade common femoral artery approach: factors associated with access time. *J. Vasc. Access.* 15: 1129729820942053.

23 Yeow, K.-M., Toh, C.-H., Wu, C.-H. et al. (2002). Sonographically guided antegrade common femoral artery access. *J. Ultrasound. Med.* 21 (12): 1413–1416.

24 Micari, A., Brodmann, M., Keirse, K. et al. (2018). Drug-coated balloon treatment of femoropopliteal lesions for patients with intermittent claudication and ischemic rest pain: 2-year results from the IN.PACT global study. *JACC Cardiovasc. Interv.* 11 (10): 945–953.

25 Kokkinidis, D.G., Jeon-Slaughter, H., Khalili, H. et al. (2018). Adjunctive stent use during endovascular intervention to the femoropopliteal artery with drug coated balloons: insights from the XLPAD registry. *Vasc. Med.* 23 (4): 358–364.

26 Horie, K., Tanaka, A., Taguri, M. et al. (2018). Impact of prolonged inflation times during plain balloon angioplasty on angiographic dissection in femoropopliteal lesions. *J. Endovasc. Ther.* 25 (6): 683–691.

27 Armstrong, E.J., Brodmann, M., Deaton, D.H. et al. (2019). Dissections after infrainguinal percutaneous transluminal angioplasty: a systematic review and current state of clinical evidence. *J. Endovasc. Ther.* 26 (4): 479–489.

28 Feldman, D.N., Armstrong, E.J., Aronow, H.D. et al. (2018). SCAI consensus guidelines for device selection in femoral-popliteal arterial interventions. *Catheter. Cardiovasc. Interv.* 92 (1): 124–140.

29 Canaud, L., Alric, P., Berthet, J.-P. et al. (2008). Infrainguinal cutting balloon angioplasty in de novo arterial lesions. *J. Vasc. Surg.* 48 (5): 1182–1188.

30 Mustapha, J.A., Lansky, A., Shishehbor, M. et al. (2018). A prospective, multi-center study of the chocolate balloon in femoropopliteal peripheral artery disease: the chocolate BAR registry. *Catheter. Cardiovasc. Interv.* 91: 1144–1148. http://dx.doi.org/10.1002/ccd.27565.

31 Adams, G., Shammas, N., Mangalmurti, S. et al. (2020). Intravascular lithotripsy for treatment of calcified lower extremity arterial stenosis: initial analysis of the disrupt PAD III study. *J. Endovasc. Ther.* 27 (3): 473–480.

32 Katsanos, K., Kitrou, P., Spiliopoulos, S. et al. (2016). Comparative effectiveness of plain balloon angioplasty, bare metal stents, drug-coated balloons, and drug-eluting stents for the treatment of infrapopliteal artery disease. *J. Endovasc. Therap.* 23: 851–863. http://dx.doi.org/10.1177/1526602816671740.

33 Katsanos, K., Spiliopoulos, S., Kitrou, P. et al. (2018). Risk of death following application of paclitaxel-coated balloons and stents in the femoropopliteal artery of the leg: a systematic review and meta-analysis of randomized controlled trials. *J. Am. Heart Assoc.* 7 (24): e011245.

34 Nordanstig, J., James, S., Andersson, M. et al. (2020). Mortality with paclitaxel-coated devices in peripheral artery disease. *N. Engl. J. Med.* 383 (26): 2538–2546.

35 Finn, M.T., Ingrassia, J.J., and Parikh, S.A. (2020). Plaque modification in endovascular patients with infrainguinal procedures. *Interventional Cardiology Clinics* 9 (2): 125.

36 Dave, R.M., Patlola, R., Kollmeyer, K. et al. (2009). Excimer laser recanalization of femoropopliteal lesions and 1-year patency: results of the CELLO registry. *J. Endovasc. Ther.* 16 (6): 665–675.

37 Dippel, E.J., Makam, P., Kovach, R. et al. (2015). Randomized controlled study of excimer laser atherectomy for treatment of femoropopliteal in-stent restenosis: initial results from the EXCITE ISR trial (EXCImer Laser Randomized Controlled Study for Treatment of FemoropopliTEal In-Stent Restenosis). *JACC Cardiovasc. Interv.* 8 (1 Part A): 92–101.

38 Henry, M., Amor, M., Ethevenot, G. et al. (1995). Percutaneous peripheral atherectomy using the rotablator: a single-center experience. *J. Endovasc. Surg.* 2 (1): 51–66.

39 Gray, W.A., Garcia, L.A., Amin, A. et al. (2018). Jetstream atherectomy system treatment of femoropopliteal arteries: results of the post-market JET registry. *Cardiovasc. Revasc. Med.* 19 (5 Pt A): 506–511.

40 Shammas, N.W., Shammas, G.A., Jones-Miller, S. et al. (2018). Long-term outcomes with Jetstream atherectomy with or without drug coated balloons in treating femoropopliteal arteries: a single center experience (JET-SCE). *Cardiovasc. Revasc. Med.* 19 (7 Pt A): 771–777.

41 Davis, T., Ramaiah, V., Niazi, K. et al. (2017). Safety and effectiveness of the phoenix atherectomy system in lower extremity arteries: early and midterm outcomes from the prospective multicenter EASE study. *Vascular* 25 (6): 563–575.

42 Rodoplu, O., Oztas, D.M., Meric, M. et al. (2020). Efficacy of rotational atherectomy followed by drug-coated balloon angioplasty for the treatment of femoropopliteal lesions-comparison with sole drug-coated balloon revascularization: two-year outcomes. *Ann. Vasc. Surg.* https://europepmc.org/article/med/33359329.

43 Charitakis, K. and Feldman, D.N. (2015). Atherectomy for lower extremity intervention: why, when, and which device? American College of Cardiology.

44 McKinsey, J.F., Zeller, T., Rocha-Singh, K.J. et al. (2014). Lower extremity revascularization using directional atherectomy: 12-month prospective results of the DEFINITIVE LE study. *JACC Cardiovasc. Interv.* 7 (8): 923–933.

45 Zeller, T., Langhoff, R., Rocha-Singh, K.J. et al. (2017). Directional atherectomy followed by a paclitaxel-coated balloon to inhibit restenosis and maintain vessel patency: twelve-month results of the DEFINITIVE AR study. *Circ. Cardiovasc. Interv.* 10 (9): http://dx.doi.org/10.1161/CIRCINTERVENTIONS.116.004848.

46 Schwindt, A.G., Bennett, J.G. Jr., Crowder, W.H. et al. (2017). Lower extremity revascularization using optical coherence tomography-guided directional atherectomy: final results of the EvaluatIon of the PantheriS OptIcal Coherence Tomography ImagiNg Atherectomy system for use in the peripheral vasculature (VISION) study. *J. Endovasc. Ther.* 24 (3): 355–366.

47 Dattilo, R., Himmelstein, S.I., and Cuff, R.F. (2014). The COMPLIANCE 360 trial: a randomized, prospective, multicenter, pilot study comparing acute and long-term results of orbital atherectomy to balloon angioplasty for calcified femoropopliteal disease. *J. Invasive Cardiol.* 26 (8): 355–360.

48 Bhatt, H., Kovach, R., Janzer, S., and George, J.C. (2018). SUPERA stent outcomes in Above-The-Knee IntervEntions: effects of COMPression and Elongation (SAKE-COMPEL) sub-study. *Cardiovasc. Revasc. Med.* 19 (5 Pt A): 512–515.

49 Park, S.H., SENS-FP Investigators, Rha, S.W. et al. (2014). Efficacy of two different self-expanding nitinol stents for atherosclerotic femoropopliteal arterial disease (SENS-FP trial): study protocol for a randomized controlled trial. *Trials* 15: http://dx.doi.org/10.1186/1745-6215-15-355.

50 Garcia, L.A., Rosenfield, K.R., Metzger, C.D. et al. (2017). SUPERB final 3-year outcomes using interwoven nitinol biomimetic supera stent. *Catheter. Cardiovasc. Interv.* 89: 1259–1267. http://dx.doi.org/10.1002/ccd.27058.

51 Ni, Q., Yang, S., Xue, G. et al. (2020). Viabahn stent graft for the endovascular treatment of occlusive lesions in the femoropopliteal artery: a retrospective cohort study with 4-year follow-up. *Ann. Vasc. Surg.* 66: 573–579.

10

Tibial Interventions in Patients with Critical Limb-Threatening Ischemia

Raman Sharma[1], Roberto Cerrud-Rodriguez[2], and Prakash Krishnan[1]

[1] Division of Cardiology, The Zena and Michael A. Weiner Cardiovascular Institute, Icahn School of Medicine at Mount Sinai, New York, NY, USA
[2] Division of Cardiology, Albert Einstein College of Medicine-Montefiore Medical Center, Bronx, NY, USA

Introduction

Critical limb-threatening ischemia (CLTI) is the clinical syndrome of ischemic rest pain, ulcer, or gangrene due to ischemic peripheral arterial disease supported by hemodynamic criteria [1]. The distinction is made from acute limb ischemia, which is defined as <14 days, and takes several weeks to months [2]. Patients presenting with CLTI are classified as Rutherford Stage ≥4 or Fontaine Stage III/IV (Table 10.1).

Morbidity and mortality for patients presenting with CLTI is largely determined by their elevated cardiovascular events [4–6]. One-year risk of myocardial infarction and stroke in CLTI patients ranges from 30 to 50%, which is same risk that all peripheral arterial disease (PAD) patients are exposed to over a five-year period [6–8]. Similarly, patients with CLTI without revascularization have a 30–50% risk of major amputation (at or above the ankle) [9].

Indications and Goals of Endovascular Revascularization

The majority of CLTI patients can be offered an endovascular, surgical, or hybrid approach to revascularization as opposed to upfront amputation [1, 9–11]. It is important to identify the patients who will warrant primary amputation through thorough history, physical examination with respects to paresis, ulcer/gangrene

Endovascular Interventions: A Step-by-Step Approach, First Edition. Edited by Jose M. Wiley, Cristina Sanina, George D. Dangas, and Prakash Krishnan.
© 2023 John Wiley & Sons Ltd. Published 2023 by John Wiley & Sons Ltd.

Table 10.1 Classification, staging and clinical symptoms of intermittent claudication and chronic limb-threatening ischemia [1, 3].

	Symptom	Rutherford classification	Fontaine classification
Intermittent claudication	Asymptomatic	Stage 0	Stage I
	Mild claudication	Stage 1	Stage IIA (Symptoms after >200 m)
	Moderate claudication	Stage 2	Stage IIB (Symptoms before <200 m)
	Severe claudication	Stage 3	
Critical limb-threatening ischemia	Ischemic rest pain	Stage 4	Stage III
	Minor ulceration	Stage 5	Stage IV
	Major ulceration or gangrene	Stage 6	

characteristics, life expectancy, and overall functionality. Classifications systems, such as the WIfI classification (**W**ound, **I**schemia, Foot **I**nfection), can be used to help estimate a patients one-year risk of amputation as well as the benefit of/requirement for revascularization [12–14].

For the CLTI patients undergoing revascularization, the goals of intervention can be generalized into the following [1]:

1) Alleviation of ischemic rest pain
2) Wound healing (both presenting wounds and primary amputation sites)
3) Improve physical functionality of affected limb

The endovascular approach to revascularization for CLTI is a less invasive strategy when compared to surgical approach [15]. It should be taken into consideration that the endovascular approach is known to be less durable when compared to the surgical approach [16]. This may not, however, be a key element in the decision-making process when considering the goal of allowing for wound healing along with the overall life expectancy of the CLTI population. In patients with better functional status, longer life expectancy, and an adequate endogenous vein for grafting, the morbidity associated with surgical revascularization may be outweighed by longer term benefits of lower reintervention rates and overall improved durability [15–17].

Considerations for Access Site

An early decision to make in approaching endovascular revascularization of patients presenting with CLTI is the access site. Below are the most common access sites to be used [18–20]:

1) Contralateral retrograde CFA access for antegrade intervention

2) Ipsilateral antegrade CFA/SFA access for antegrade intervention
3) Distal tibial artery retrograde access for retrograde intervention ± contralateral/ipsilateral CFA access

We recommend that initial access for revascularization should be the contralateral CFA for antegrade intervention. Alternative access should be considered with extreme iliac tortuosity, hostile groins, prior EVAR with iliac limbs, common iliac artery stents with neocarina formation, aortofemoral bypass, need for considerable support for successful crossing, and available device lengths in very tall patients.

When considering ipsilateral antegrade CFA/SFA access, attention should be made to the available vessel length for the sheath (i.e. a proximal SFA lesion will make it challenging for successful delivery of sheath). Vascular complications are increased with antegrade access, particularly in obese patients [21].

Tibial access is also an option for access in CLTI intervention, when used as a sole access (transpedal arterial minimally invasive [TAMI] retrograde revascularization), or in conjunction with proximal access for lesion crossing, wire externalization, and subsequent antegrade intervention [22]. Access can be made with smaller diameter sheaths, even sheathless access, which is particularly useful when used as a means of lesion crossing and wire externalization [23].

Single Versus Multitibial Artery Revascularization

An additional decision to make when planning tibial revascularization for CLTI is whether intervention should be limited to a single tibial artery or multiple. An important concept to mention in this debate is that of angiosomes [24]. According to the classic study by Taylor and Palmer [25] an angiosome is a three-dimensional unit of tissue in the lower extremity, considered unique vascular territory supplied by source arteries and veins. Based on this theory, the location of the ulcer, depending on the affected angiosome (Figure 10.1), should be guide the intervention towards the single target vessel responsible for its circulation [25–28].

However, there seems to be contradictory data as in some studies, angiosome-driven single tibial artery revascularization resulted in improvement in skin perfusion pressures with only a 50% angiosome correlation [29]. Moreover, a recent study by Kurianov et al. showed no significant difference in outcomes in patients with CTLI secondary to multilevel PAD treated with angiosome-guided (direct, targeting the artery supplying the ischemic wound) revascularization vs. those treated with non-angiosomic (indirect, targeting an artery supplying collaterals to the ischemic wound) revascularization [30].

Multitibial intervention has been shown to promote improved wound healing and faster healing times when compared with single tibial intervention [31]. It must be noted, however, that unaccounted confounders might exist that could potentially influence the results of these studies.

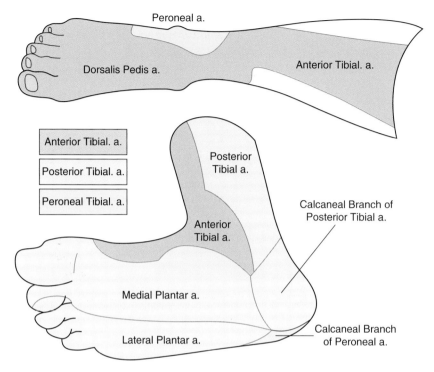

Figure 10.1 Angiosomes. This figure illustrates the concept of the angiosomes as units of tissue in the foot receiving irrigation from a specific artery.

Antegrade Tibial Artery Intervention

Once the target vessel for intervention has been identified, one can begin the intervention. In regard to selecting the sheath, almost every tibial intervention can be successfully completed with a 6 Fr system, some through even smaller sizes. It is imperative to have adequate digital subtraction angiography images for reference or roadmap when wiring long tibial lesions, especially long CTO segments (Figure 10.2). This can be accomplished through imaging directly from the popliteal artery with a 0.035″ catheter or through the tibial vessel in question with a 0.018″ catheter (injection through a 0.014″ catheter may prove very challenging and provide poor images).

Once the appropriate images have been obtained, it is important to carefully analyze the images for channels of native lumen, CTO segments, and islands of native vessel in between. If a microchannel is present, an 0.014″ hydrophilic tip wire (e.g., Command, Fielder, Ficlder XT, etc.) with a 0.014″ or 0.018″ microcatheter (e.g., Teleport, TrailBlazer, etc.) can be used first. Advancing the wire, torquing frequently to avoid small collateral branches, often is quite simple when a

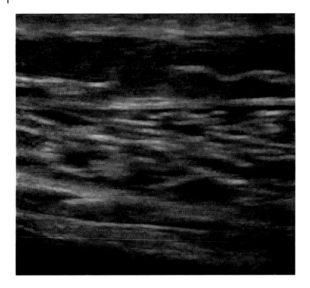

Figure 10.2   Wire inside a tibial vessel. This figure demonstrates the appearance of a guidewire inside one of the tibial vessels, as seen using ultrasound. The red arrows help identify the guidewire.

channel is available. The catheter should be advanced over the wire to the distal tibial/pedal vessel and the wire should be exchanged for a workhorse wire that does not have a hydrophilic tip to avoid unnecessary complications (e.g., SpartaCore, Runthrough, etc.) It is good practice to take a small injection of contrast through the catheter once in the pedal circulation to confirm location within lumen, making sure to draw back blood first.

Once the wire has been exchanged, balloon angioplasty, preceded by atherectomy or atherotomy, should be performed. Directional atherectomy or orbital atherectomy are the most common modalities, and both are done over an 0.014″ wire. Adequate vasodilators should be administered to limit significant downstream embolization. We recommend that balloon angioplasty be performed with 1:1 balloons to avoid dissections of the vessel that would require stenting. Final DSA imaging should be taken again after vasodilator administration to demonstrate patent tibial post intervention.

Tibial CTO lesions requiring revascularization pose an additional challenge and unfortunately are more commonly found in the CLTI population; we recommend DSA imaging through catheters to optimize the anatomic information obtained through imaging. In our experience, a trial of a hydrophilic wire is not unreasonable as a first attempt, although in CTO lesions this will likely be unsuccessful. Two main issues will be confronted when traversing the CTO: (a) lesion crossing with CTO wire and (b) lack of support. Regarding wires, traditional coronary CTO wires can be used to cross the lesion (e.g., Confianza, Confianza Pro, Astato, etc.) and escalated appropriately. Often as the wire makes forward progress, the lack of support becomes an evolving problem, especially in the setting of a heavily calcific vessel and multiple caps requiring penetration. Given the overall complexity in crossing, an 0.014″ microcatheter (e.g., Teleport, Corsair, etc.) is a better choice over an 0.018″ catheter. Effort should be made consistently advance the microcatheter to provide additional support to allow for further advancing of the wire. Corkscrewing/push-pulling and other techniques should be performed to advance the microcatheter as needed.

In the event the microcatheter is unable to be advanced, several options are available. First, the microcatheter can be exchanged for another. For example, if the Teleport is used first, exchanging it for Corsair, which has a lower tip entry profile (1.3 Fr vs 1.4 Fr) and a braided pattern that allows for corkscrewing the microcatheter forward, may allow for crossing of the microcatheter over the lesion. Another option is to withdraw the microcatheter and begin balloon dilatation with short, small diameter coronary balloons (1.0 mm, 1.5 mm, 2.0 mm). This may help the subsequent delivery of the microcatheter. Finally, a guide extension catheter may be used and advanced to the tibial vessel, and all of these steps can be repeated until success. Once the lesion has been traversed, atherectomy/atherotomy and balloon angioplasty should be performed, again with copious amounts of vasodilators.

In the event that none of these techniques prove successful, one can try dissection-reentry, also known as **S**ubintimal **T**racking **A**nd **R**eentry (STAR) technique [32], before pursuing retrograde access. Care should be taken to ensure the dissection flap created is always small. Reentry can be performed by pushing the knuckle directly into the lumen, which may be challenging and require the use of CTO wires, reentry devices or angled microcatheters, among other tools. Orbital atherectomy should be avoided when approaching the treatment of peripheral CTO using a subintimal approach due to the risk of extending the dissection plane across the ostia of important side vessels [33].

Retrograde Access for Retrograde Lesion Crossing and Wire Externalization with Antegrade Revascularization

It is important to continue to consider fluoroscopy time, radiation, and contrast use in these complex CLTI cases. When struggling with antegrade for a long time, it is a reasonable strategy to adjust the approach to include a retrograde access to facilitate lesion crossing for subsequent antegrade revascularization [33]. In this approach, the retrograde approach is solely performed to allow for retrograde lesion crossing and wire externalization; the lesion is not treated in a retrograde fashion but rather still antegrade.

Since there is no plan for intervention from the retrograde approach, the access sheath can be as small as a 2.9 F, 4 F or even a sheath less approach. Access should be obtained near the ankle with ultrasound guidance as well as fluoroscopic guidance, with a standard 21-gauge micro access needle and a 0.014″ or 0.018″ wire. Depending on the plan for retrograde lesion crossing, the choice of access site sheath, or lack thereof, should be made. This is dependent on the available equipment as well as the planned retrograde crossing technique.

Regarding crossing techniques, coronary retrograde CTO crossing techniques have been adopted in peripheral CTO crossing, specifically in tibial CTOs. The most performed are the **S**ubintimal **A**rterial **F**lossing with **A**ntegrade-- **R**etrograde **I**ntervention (SAFARI) [34], **C**ontrolled **A**ntegrade and **R**etrograde **T**racking (CART) [35], and **R**everse **C**ontrolled **A**ntegrade and **R**etrograde **T**racking (Reverse CART) [36]. The SAFARI technique involves the creation of both antegrade and retrograde dissections in the subintimal space with the goal of having the wires connect the planes at some level. Once the wires are interacting in a unified plane, the retrograde wire can be externalized, or flossed, through the lesion to now allow for antegrade intervention [34]. CART can be considered a controlled modification of SAFARI. In CART, an antegrade dissection is created and a balloon is inflated within the subintimal space. The retrograde wire is then directed into this space in order to then be externalized and subsequent antegrade intervention [35]. The reverse of this (reverse CART) simply refers to the subintimal dissection and balloon inflation be created by the retrograde approach, whereby the antegrade wire is directed into the subintimal space and into the distal vessel lumen, followed by antegrade intervention [36].

TAMI Retrograde Revascularization

A mention should be made for TAMI retrograde revascularization. In certain scenarios, it may be feasible to perform the entire intervention solely from the pedal access. Orbital atherectomy can be performed through a 4 Fr system; as long as the wire transit remains transluminal, it is a atherectomy device that can potentially be used. Balloon delivery is also not as issue as these devices also can be utilized over a 4 Fr system. Directional atherectomy, on the other hand, is not available from the pedal approach as it requires a 6 Fr system.

Although the concept to total revascularization from the pedal access sounds intriguing, it is imperative that the operator judiciously choose the cases in which this is an appropriate approach (Figure 10.3), for several reasons. CLTI patients are by a vast majority diabetic patients, all of whom have uniquely diseased tibial

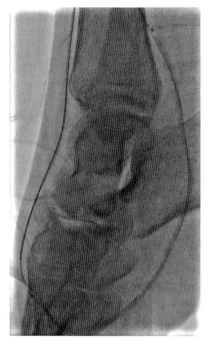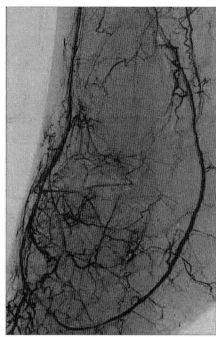

Figure 10.3 Crossing of a CTO of the lateral plantar artery with subsequent crossing of a CTO of the posterior tibial artery. The left panel illustrates the sequential wiring of the anterior pedal and dorsalis pedis artery, followed by the crossing of a CTO of the lateral plantar artery and of a subsequent CTO of the posterior tibial artery. The right panel shows the reconstitution of flow after balloon angioplasty (not shown).

anatomy. Access site dissection and thrombus are serious concerns in these patients, especially when the sheath itself may be occlusive so the diagnosis of these consequences can potentially be delayed. Bailout options are also lacking from the retrograde approach. Balloon tamponade may be performed, but most coronary stents and all covered stents will not fit through a 4 Fr sheath, should they be needed.

It is our opinion that a reasonable patient for TAMI retrograde revascularization would be one with a patent tibial vessel around the ankle and with a lesion that appears to be of low complexity that can be successfully crossed transluminally. Appropriate patient selection will aim towards the highest chance at success from the pedal approach while minimizing complications. As of now, data is still lacking in success, access site related injury, and best practices for pedal access intervention, but as the field continues to evolve these questions will be answered with future studies.

Reentry and Externalization Devices

For tibial interventions, the only available reentry device is the Enteer Re-entry Balloon Catheter [37] that has a specific below the knee model. This 5 Fr compatible flat-shaped balloon is 0.014″ or 0.018″ wire compatible that orients itself to the true lumen when inflated. The Enteer guidewires are then advanced through the device towards the exit port and puncture into the true lumen. The Quick-Cross Capture Guidewire Catheter is a 6 Fr, up to 0.035″ wire compatible device that can be used to aid in the process of wire externalization, as an antegrade balloon centered retrograde funnel catheter. The device is centered within the vessel with low pressure balloon inflation via the antegrade approach, which allows for easy externalization of the retrograde wire through the funnel of the device.

Deep Venous Arterialization (DVA)

In the CLTI population, especially the Rutherford Class 6 and Fontaine Stage IV, it is not uncommon to simply have no reasonable target for revascularization. In the setting of the "desert foot," a major amputation upfront is a reasonable strategy [38]. Recently, however, there has been a new technique with the goal of avoiding, or at least delaying, major amputation. Deep venous arterialization is a technique in which a patent proximal tibial artery and vein are fistulized with a covered stent to supply oxygenated blood to the foot through venous circulation [39].

Our approach is as follows: antegrade access is taken as usual and pedal vein access is taken as well. The latter access is again taken with ultrasound guidance and micropuncture technique. Advancing the wire through the vein will at times be obstructed due to venous valves but torquing the wire should allow for advancement. The pedal access can be sheathless again, but can be upgraded to a 6 Fr slender sheath if necessary. For creating the fistula, the Outback Elite Re-Entry Catheter [40] or the Pioneer Plus IVUS Guided Re-Entry Catheter [41] should be used. Once the antegrade wire has been advanced to the venous system, the creating of the fistula can be performed with covered stents, either coronary or peripheral depending on the appropriate size requirements. Once the fistula is created, if an angiogram is taken it will appear as though there is no flow into the foot, which is the result of the venous valves and these need to be treated as well. Fracturing the valves with atherotomy balloons and stenting with covered stents are the typical steps for preparing the venous circulation for the arterialized flow. Any prominent collateral branches of the tibial vein will also require covered stenting as to ensure the arterial flow is directed to the foot through a single vessel. These can be better visualized with contrast injection in the distal tibial vein and identification of the significant collaterals. Once all these steps are completed a final angiogram should show antegrade blood flow directly from the patent tibial artery all the way through the venous arch.

A few key points must be considered: these patients will still undergo amputation, but hopefully it will be limited to a minor amputation. Moreover, prior to pursuing this revascularization strategy, it must be ensured that the patient has an intact venous arch in the foot. Without this, the DVA may ultimately prove to be ineffective [42]. By creating the fistula from the artery to the vein, the distal venous circulation requires 6–8 weeks to mature be able to appropriately accommodate the arterialized blood flow. The minor amputation should be performed at that time. A common complain after a successful procedure is a sensation of fullness in the effected limb, which is a direct result of the arterial blood flow within the venous system, and of which patients must be educated about beforehand to avoid unnecessary emotional distress.

References

1 Conte, M.S., Bradbury, A.W., Kolh, P. et al. (2019). Global vascular guidelines on the management of chronic limb-threatening ischemia. *J. Vasc. Surg.* 69 (6, Supplement): 3S–125S.e40.

2 Ruiz-Carmona, C., Clara, A., Casajuana, E. et al. (2022). Clinical Clues for the Current Diagnosis of Acute Lower Limb Ischemia: A Contemporary Case Series. *Ann. Vasc. Surg.* 79: 174–181.

3 McDermott, M.M., Greenland, P., Liu, K. et al. (2001). Leg symptoms in peripheral arterial disease: associated clinical characteristics and functional impairment. *JAMA* 286 (13): 1599–1606.

4 Smith, G.D., Shipley, M.J., and Rose, G. (1990). Intermittent claudication, heart disease risk factors, and mortality. The Whitehall Study. *Circulation* 82 (6): 1925–1931.

5 Smith, F.B., Rumley, A., Lee, A.J. et al. (1998). Haemostatic factors and prediction of ischaemic heart disease and stroke in claudicants. *Br. J. Haematol.* 100 (4): 758–763.

6 Norgren, L., Hiatt, W.R., Dormandy, J.A. et al. (2007). Inter-Society Consensus for the Management of Peripheral Arterial Disease (TASC II). *J. Vasc. Surg.* 45 (Suppl S): S5–S67.

7 Gerhard-Herman, M.D., Gornik, H.L., Barrett, C. et al. (2017). 2016 AHA/ACC Guideline on the Management of Patients With Lower Extremity Peripheral Artery Disease: A Report of the American College of Cardiology/American Heart Association Task Force on Clinical Practice Guidelines. *Circulation* 135 (12): e726–e779.

8 Davies, M.G. (2012). Criticial limb ischemia: epidemiology. *Methodist Debakey Cardiovasc. J.* 8 (4): 10–14.

9 Aboyans, V., Ricco, J.B., Bartelink, M.E.L. et al. (2018). 2017 ESC Guidelines on the Diagnosis and Treatment of Peripheral Arterial Diseases, in collaboration with the European Society for Vascular Surgery (ESVS): Document covering atherosclerotic disease of extracranial carotid and vertebral, mesenteric, renal, upper and lower extremity arteriesEndorsed by: the European Stroke Organization (ESO)The Task Force for the Diagnosis and Treatment of Peripheral Arterial Diseases of the European Society of Cardiology (ESC) and of the European Society for Vascular Surgery (ESVS). *Eur. Heart J.* 39 (9): 763–816.

10 Stella, J., Engelbertz, C., Gebauer, K. et al. (2019). Outcome of patients with chronic limb-threatening ischemia with and without revascularization. *Vasa* 49 (2): 121–127.

11 Domínguez, L.J.G., Moreno, I.R., Núñez, L.G., and Hernández, M.M. (2021). Hybrid revascularization of chronic limb-threatening ischemia using popliteal below-knee and tibial trifurcation open endarterectomy distally plus inter-woven nitinol stenting proximally. *Ann. Vasc. Surg.*.

12 Cerqueira, L.O., Duarte, E.G., Barros, A.L.S. et al. (2020). WIfI classification: the Society for Vascular Surgery lower extremity threatened limb classification system, a literature review. *J. Vasc. Bras.* 19: e20190070–e.

13 Mills, J.L., Conte, M.S., Armstrong, D.G. et al. (2014). The Society for Vascular Surgery Lower Extremity Threatened Limb Classification System: Risk stratification based on Wound, Ischemia, and foot Infection (WIfI). *J. Vasc. Surg.* 59 (1): 220–34.e2.

14 Zhan, L.X., Branco, B.C., Armstrong, D.G., and Mills, J.L. Sr. (2015). The Society for Vascular Surgery lower extremity threatened limb classification system based on Wound, Ischemia, and foot Infection (WIfI) correlates with risk of major amputation and time to wound healing. *J. Vasc. Surg.* 61 (4): 939–944.

15 Parvar, S.L., Ngo, L., Dawson, J. et al. (2022). Long-term outcomes following endovascular and surgical revascularization for peripheral artery disease: a propensity score-matched analysis. *Eur. Heart J.* 43 (1): 32–40.

16 Utsunomiya, M., Takahara, M., Iida, O. et al. (2020). Limb-Based Patency After Surgical vs Endovascular Revascularization in Patients with Chronic Limb-Threatening Ischemia. *J. Endovasc. Ther.* 27 (4): 584–594.

17 Chung, J., Bartelson, B.B., Hiatt, W.R. et al. (2006). Wound healing and functional outcomes after infrainguinal bypass with reversed saphenous vein for critical limb ischemia. *J. Vasc. Surg.* 43 (6): 1183–1190.

18 Spiliopoulos, S., Katsanos, K., Karnabatidis, D. et al. (2011). Safety and efficacy of the StarClose vascular closure device in more than 1000 consecutive peripheral angioplasty procedures. *J. Endovasc. Ther.* 18 (3): 435–443.

19 Ruzsa, Z., Nemes, B., Bánsághi, Z. et al. (2014). Transpedal access after failed anterograde recanalization of complex below-the-knee and femoropopliteal occlusions in critical limb ischemia. *Catheter. Cardiovasc. Interv.* 83 (6): 997–1007.

20 Pezold, M., Blumberg, S., Sadek, M. et al. (2021). Antegrade Superficial Femoral Artery Access for Lower Extremity Arterial Disease Is Safe and Effective in the Outpatient Setting. *Ann. Vasc. Surg.* 72: 175–181.

21 Wheatley, B.J., Mansour, M.A., Grossman, P.M. et al. (2011). Complication rates for percutaneous lower extremity arterial antegrade access. *Arch. Surg.* 146 (4): 432–435.

22 Mustapha, J.A., Saab, F., McGoff, T.N. et al. (2020). Tibiopedal arterial minimally invasive retrograde revascularization (TAMI) in patients with peripheral arterial disease and critical limb ischemia. On behalf of the Peripheral Registry of Endovascular Clinical Outcomes (PRIME). *Catheter. Cardiovasc. Interv.* 95 (3): 447–454.

23 El-Sayed, H.F. (2013). Retrograde pedal/tibial artery access for treatment of infragenicular arterial occlusive disease. *Methodist Debakey Cardiovasc. J.* 9 (2): 73–78.

24 Alexandrescu, V., Söderström, M., and Venermo, M. (2012). Angiosome theory: fact or fiction? *Scand. J. Surg.* 101 (2): 125–131.

25 Taylor, G.I. and Pan, W.R. (1998). Angiosomes of the leg: anatomic study and clinical implications. *Plast. Reconstr. Surg.* 102 (3): 599–616; discussion 7-8.

26 Söderström, M., Albäck, A., Biancari, F. et al. (2013). Angiosome-targeted infrapopliteal endovascular revascularization for treatment of diabetic foot ulcers. *J. Vasc. Surg.* 57 (2): 427–435.

27 Kabra, A., Suresh, K.R., Vivekanand, V. et al. (2013). Outcomes of angiosome and non-angiosome targeted revascularization in critical lower limb ischemia. *J. Vasc. Surg.* 57 (1): 44–49.

28 Yamada, T., Shibahara, T., Nagase, M. et al. (2022). Validation of the correlation between angiosome-based target arterial path, mid-term limb-based patency, and the global limb anatomical staging system. *Heart Vessel.* 37 (3): 496–504.

29 Kawarada, O., Yasuda, S., Nishimura, K. et al. (2014). Effect of Single Tibial Artery Revascularization on Microcirculation in the Setting of Critical Limb Ischemia. *Circ. Cardiovasc. Interv.* 7 (5): 684–691.

30 Kurianov, P., Lipin, A., Antropov, A. et al. (2022). Propensity-matched analysis does not support angiosome-guided revascularization of multilevel peripheral artery disease (PAD). *Vasc. Med.* 27 (1): 47–54.

31 Kobayashi, N., Hirano, K., Yamawaki, M. et al. (2017). Clinical effects of single or double tibial artery revascularization in critical limb ischemia patients with tissue loss. *J. Vasc. Surg.* 65 (3): 744–753.

32 Colombo, A., Mikhail, G.W., Michev, I. et al. (2005). Treating chronic total occlusions using subintimal tracking and reentry: the STAR technique. *Catheter. Cardiovasc. Interv.* 64 (4): 407–411; discussion 12.

33 Sheeran, D. and Wilkins, L.R. (2018). Long Chronic Total Occlusions: Revascularization Strategies. *Semin. Interv. Radiol.* 35 (5): 469–476.

34 Phadke, D.R., Sheeran, D., Angle, J., and Wilkins, L. (2020). Application of the gunsight technique to facilitate subintimal arterial flossing with antegrade-retrograde intervention for the treatment of lower extremity chronic total occlusion. *Am. J. Interv. Radiol.* 4: 12.

35 Igari, K., Kudo, T., Toyofuku, T., and Inoue, Y. (2015). Controlled antegrade and retrograde subintimal tracking technique for endovascular treatment of the superficial femoral artery with chronic total occlusion. *Ann. Vasc. Surg.* 29 (6): 1320.e7–e10.

36 Matsuno, S., Tsuchikane, E., Harding, S.A. et al. (2018). Overview and proposed terminology for the reverse controlled antegrade and retrograde tracking (reverse CART) techniques. *EuroIntervention* 14 (1): 94–101.

37 Wosik, J., Shorrock, D., Christopoulos, G. et al. (2015). Systematic Review of the BridgePoint System for Crossing Coronary and Peripheral Chronic Total Occlusions. *J. Invasive Cardiol.* 27 (6): 269–276.

38 Kim, T.I., Vartanian, S.S., and Schneider, P.A. (2021). A Review and Proposed Classification System for the No-Option Patient With Chronic Limb-Threatening Ischemia. *J. Endovasc. Ther.* 28 (2): 183–193.

39 N'Dandu, Z., Bonilla, J., Yousef, G.M., and White, C.J. (2021). Percutaneous deep vein arterialization: An emerging technique for no-option chronic limb-threatening ischemia patients. *Catheter. Cardiovasc. Interv.* 97 (4): 685–690.

40 Hayakawa, N., Kodera, S., Arakawa, M., and Kanda, J. (2020). Successful re-entry using the outback® elite catheter via retrograde popliteal access with IVUS guidance for femoropopliteal occlusion: a case report. *CVIR Endovasc.* 3 (1): 63.

41 Saketkhoo, R.R., Razavi, M.K., Padidar, A. et al. (2004). Percutaneous bypass: subintimal recanalization of peripheral occlusive disease with IVUS guided luminal re-entry. *Tech. Vasc. Interv. Radiol.* 7 (1): 23–27.

42 Kum, S., Tan, Y.K., Schreve, M.A. et al. (2017). Midterm Outcomes From a Pilot Study of Percutaneous Deep Vein Arterialization for the Treatment of No-Option Critical Limb Ischemia. *J. Endovasc. Ther.* 24 (5): 619–626.

11

Acute Limb Ischemia

Endovascular Approach

Shunsuke Aoi[1] and Amit M. Kakkar[2]

[1] *Division of Cardiology, Albert Einstein College of Medicine-Montefiore Medical Center, Bronx, NY, USA*
[2] *Division of Cardiology, Albert Einstein College of Medicine-Jacobi Medical Center, Bronx, NY, USA*

Introduction

Acute limb ischemia (ALI) is defined as a sudden decrease in limb perfusion that threatens the viability of the limb. ALI is a vascular emergency and delay in diagnosis and management place patients at risk for limb loss and adverse events. Multiple endovascular techniques are now suitable to deal with this critical issue. Many endovascular suites carry an array of devices which can be used to treat acute limb patients. Catheter-directed thrombolysis has emerged as the treatment of choice for many patients with threatened but salvageable limb with no contraindications to thrombolysis. We review the key steps to the management of this potentially life-threatening clinical condition.

Procedure Planning, Equipment, and Considerations

Step 1. Diagnostic Angiography

Once the diagnosis of ALI is made, anticoagulation with intravenous heparin (goal PTT 60–80) should be initiated as soon as possible to prevent propagation of thrombus. Access site is obtained, which is often the contralateral common femoral artery of the affected limb. If available, initial diagnostic imaging to correctly identify the location of the occlusion and distal runoff is crucial in procedure planning. Commonly, aortoiliac angiography is obtained to identify any potential aortoiliac disease as a source of embolization as well as assessing the difficulty of catheter manipulation depending on the tortuosity, calcification, or narrow bifurcation angle. Subsequently, dedicated lower-extremity angiography of the affected limb is obtained after "up and over" technique using support or guide catheter to identify the nature of occlusion. The length of the occlusion, collateral channels, distal reconstitution, as well as runoff vessels should be delineated. Appropriate guide sheath size should be chosen once the affected iliofemoral anatomy is known. Typically, a minimum of 5 Fr sheath is needed for lysis devices and larger sheaths are needed for thrombectomy devices.

Tip: Carefully, assess iliac anatomy for preexisting lesions or tortuosity as guiding sheaths may move and dissect if an extended overnight procedure is required.

Step 2. Crossing the Lesion

Depending on the nature and chronicity of the occlusion (Figure 11.1), thoughtful choice of the sheath length and support catheter can maximize the chance of crossing the lesion.

Initial approach can be using the hydrophilic guidewire, such as Glidewire (Terumo, Tokyo, Japan) or Aquatrack (Cordis, Fremont, CA, USA), to probe the lesion and "knuckling" of these guidewires allow for increased push while maintaining position within the vessel architecture. Successive wire escalation to guidewires

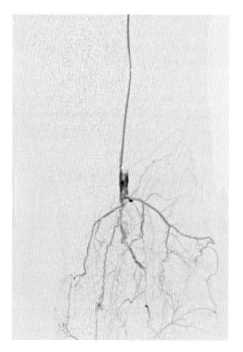

Figure 11.1 Acute thrombus of popliteal, note hazy white appearance.

with higher tipload may be necessary for occlusions with organized thrombus and underlying calcification. If unable to traverse the occlusion, thrombolytic agent administered through an endhole catheter can be considered to soften the proximal fibrin plug to increase the chance of crossing the occlusion after several hours.

Tip: When wiring, a "soft" or "butter" feel to wire advancement strongly suggest acute, fresh thrombus.

Step 3. Thrombus Management

Thrombus management can be divided into two components: thrombolysis administration and mechanical adjunct therapy.

Thrombolytic administration can significantly modify the thrombus, especially in a long segment with significant thrombus burden. Types of thrombolytic agents are listed in Table 11.1. Alteplase® is the most commonly used agent, which can be administered through a sidehole infusion catheter, such as Uni-Fuse™ catheter (Angiodynamics, Queensbury, NY, USA) or EKOS™ catheter (BTG Interventional Medicine, London, UK) (Figure 11.2), that spans the length of the occlusion to evenly distribute the medication. An array of infusion catheters are currently available (Table 11.2). There is no standardized protocol for the dose and duration of thrombolysis administration and vary significantly across the institution. Commonly, an initial bolus dose is given upfront through the sidehole infusion catheter (i.e. 2–5 mg), followed by a low-dose infusion (i.e. 0.5–1.0 mg/h fixed dose). There is no consensus on heparin use during thrombolytic infusion and risk of bleeding increases with therapeutic dose of heparin. Subtherapeutic dose of heparin may be acceptable to be infused through the sheath to prevent peri-catheter thrombosis.

Tip: tPA dosing is highly variable for acute limb cases. Interventionalists should be aware of tPA risks and contraindications (see Tables 11.3 and 11.4).

Patient should be carefully monitored for bleeding complications and blood test should be repeated to follow the level of fibrinogen and partial thromboplastin time.

Tip: Consider reducing or stopping tPA infusion if fibrinogen drops <150 or by 50% of baseline values.

1) Types of mechanical adjunct therapies to thrombolysis are listed in Table 11.5. These devices may also be considered when thrombolytic therapy is contraindicated to minimize the thrombus burden. Given the risk of distal embolization, especially in the setting of high thrombus burden and compromised distal runoff vasculature, embolic protection devices may be considered to avoid jeopardizing the distal vascular bed (Table 11.6).

Table 11.1 tPA agents (US FDA approved).

Generic name	Abbreviation	Brand name	Company	Half-life	Clearance	Initial dose	Infusion duration	Total dose
Alteplase	tPA	Activase® Cathflo activase®	Genentech	<5 min	Hepatic	2–5 mg	0.5–1.0 mg/h	40 mg maximum
Reteplase	RPA	Retavase®	Centocor	13–16 min	Hepatic and renal	2–5 units	0.25–0.5 units/h	20 units maximum
Tenecteplase	TNK	TNKase®	Genentech	20–24 min	Hepatic	1–5 mg	0.125–0.25 mg/h	NA

Figure 11.2 EKOS Endosonic catheter 40 cm in a patient with acute thrombotic occlusion of SFA stents.

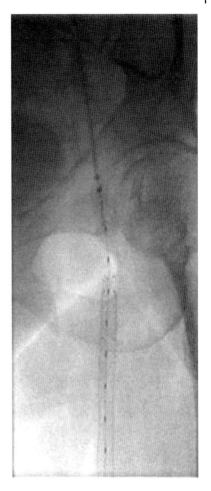

Tip: Filters can be easily deployed through 0.035″ support catheter to the desired location. To do this, place the end of the support catheter distal to the lesion and remove the wire. Insert the filter collapsed into the catheter, then advance the filter using the filter's attached wire until it emerges from the support catheter. Carefully, walk out the support catheter.

a) Aspiration thrombectomy can be performed with dual-lumen, rapid-exchange catheters such as Export® (Medtronic, Minneapolis, MN, USA) or Pronto® (Vascular Solutions, Minneapolis, MN, USA), and negative pressure created by pulling back on the syringe creates the vacuum for aspiration. Once the device is delivered proximal to the lesion, aspiration is started and continued as the catheter is advanced through the lesion. It is important to keep the suction on while pulling out to minimize the risk

Table 11.2 Commercially available infusion catheter.

Catheter	Company	Fr (Size)	Infusion/Treatment length (cm)	Shaft length (cm)	Max. wire size (inch.)	Key feature	Cons
EKOS Endosonic Mach™	BTG	6 Fr	6, 12, 18, 24, 30, 40, 50	106, 135	0.035	Ultrasound Energy, less tPA required	Cost, Bedside EKOS machine required
Uni-fuse™	Angiodynamics	4–5 Fr	2, 5, 10, 15, 20, 30, 40, 50	45, 90, 135	0.035	Multiport or endhole "drip" function	No power infusion
Cragg-McNamara™ Valved Infusion Catheter	Medtronic	4–5 Fr	5, 10, 20, 30, 40, 50	40, 65, 100, 135	0.035	Occluding ball wire	No power infusion
Fountain/Mistique®	Merit	4–5 Fr	5, 10	45, 90, 135	0.035	Forceful, pulsed injections	Multiple components

Table 11.3 tPA absolute contraindications.

tPA absolute contraindications	
1.	Prior intracranial hemorrhage
2.	Known cerebral AVMs
3.	Known cerebral neoplasm (primary or metastatic)
4.	Ischemic stroke within 3 months
5.	Suspected aortic dissection
6.	Active bleeding or bleeding diathesis
7.	Significant trauma within past 3 months

Table 11.4 tPA relative contraindications.

tPA relative contraindications	
1.	Severe uncontrolled HTN (SBP >180 mmHg or DBP >110 mmHg)
2.	Prolonged (>10 min) CPR
3.	History of prior ischemic stroke (>3 months)
4.	Major surgery <3 weeks
5.	Recent internal hemorrhage (2–4 weeks)
6.	Noncompressible vascular punctures
7.	Pregnancy
8.	Active peptic ulcer
9.	Active use of anticoagulants

Table 11.5 Mechanical adjunct to thrombolysis [1–7].

	French size	Delivery platform	Wire size (inch)	Catheter length (cm)
Aspiration				
Export	6–7 Fr	Rapid exchange	0.014	140–145
Pronto	5.5–8 Fr	Rapid exchange	0.014	138
Penumbra Indigo	3–8 Fr	Over the wire	0.035	132–150
Rheolytic				
Angiojet	4–6 Fr	Over the wire	0.014 or 0.035	90–120
Ultrasonic				
EKOS	5.4 Fr	Over the wire	0.035	106–135
Laser TurboElite/ Turbo-Tandem	4–8 Fr	Over the wire	0.014–0.035	112–150
	4–7 Fr	Rapid exchange	0.014	150

Table 11.6 Distal embolic protection devices.

Device name	Company	Sizes (mm)	Sheath size	Pore size (µm)	Pros	Cons
SpiderFx	Medtronic	3.0–6.0	6 Fr	50–200	Guidewire of choice, can use with manual or mechanical thrombectomy	Filter migration
FilterwireEZ	Boston Scientific	2.5–5.5	6 Fr	80		Must use device wire
EmboShield Nav6	Abbott	2.5–7 mm (vessel size)	5/6 Fr	140	Independently movable BareWire® can be workhouse, primary crossing wire	Must use BareWire, Difficult to deploy with tortuous vessel anatomy

of dislodging any aspirated material. It is simple to use, but the efficacy of thrombus extraction is limited due to the drop-off of vacuum created.

b) Penumbra Indigo® (Penumbra, Inc., Alameda, CA, USA) (Figure 11.3), on the other hand, allows for continuous aspiration without the drop-off of the vacuum for maximizing the aspiration power. Similarly, the device is delivered proximal to the lesion with the switch in the "off" position, then switch is turned to continuously allow aspiration as the catheter is advanced through the lesion. Separator catheter introduced inside the aspiration lumen can be used in tandem to break up the resistant thrombus during continuous aspiration. There are varieties of lineup of catheter by size; CAT8 (8 Fr) offers most efficient aspiration in the iliofemoral arteries while CAT3 (3.4 Fr) allows for treatment in the tibial arteries.

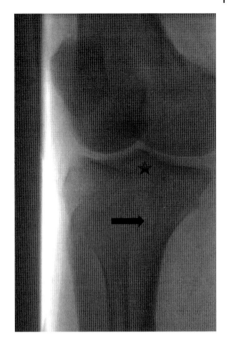

Figure 11.3 Use of Penumbra Indigo CAT3 in a patient with acute thrombus of tibial vessels. CAT3 with separator out in front (arrow).

Tip: The Indigo CAT RX® (6 Fr) is the only device in the Penumbra family that can be used on a rapid-exchange (0.014″) wire and can be used with distal embolic protection.

c) Angiojet® (Boston Scientific, Marlborough, MA, USA) rheolytic thrombectomy device is a double lumen, over the wire catheter that delivers high-pressure saline and creates a vacuum that breaks up the thrombus and suctions these fragments back out of the catheter. It can also allow delivery of tPA into the thrombus with Power Pulse™ Lytic Delivery mode to soften the organized thrombus. It is recommended to keep the device run time to less than 10 minutes to prevent excessive hemolysis, which may result in possible acute renal failure.

d) EKOS can facilitate efficacy of thrombolysis by using high-frequency ultrasound waves to accelerate thrombus dissolution. The ultrasound core wire delivers the ultrasonic waves as the thrombolytic agents are infused through the drug delivery lumen. The treatment zones can range from 6 to 50 cm, and the correct catheter should be selected from the baseline diagnostic angiography. The infusion catheter has three lumens: drug infusion port, coolant port, and main central coolant lumen. Thrombolytic agents are administered through the drug infusion port for the bolus and the continuous infusion dose of tPA. The black ultrasonic core catheter is introduced through the main central coolant lumen and screwed in at the end to be connected to the console machine.

e) Excimer laser thrombectomy delivers bursts of ultraviolet light to photoablate the lesion including thrombus, plaque, or calcium. Laser catheter should be advanced over the guidewire at a slow rate of less than 1 mm per second through the entire length of the treatment zone.

Tip: The Spectranetics Turbo-Tandem™ catheter combines a 7 Fr laser guide catheter with 2 mm excimer laser ablation catheter to create more robust treatment arc which allows for less passes. Excimer laser catheters can also be used without a wire but have difficulty navigating tortuous anatomy.

Step 4. Treating Underlying Lesion

Angiography after thrombus management can often identify the underlying lesion that contributed to the acute thrombus formation.

If the lesion appears to be amenable to conventional endovascular treatment, balloon angioplasty and/or stenting should be performed as a preferred approach. Given the extensive controversy on drug-coated balloons, the decision to use these devices should be carefully discussed with the patient and the team.

Tip: Use of a covered stent may be helpful to trap focal thrombus (or aneurysmal areas), but adequate debulking should be done first to ensure no "toothpasting" of clot distally.

Surgical revascularization may need to be discussed depending on the anatomy, thrombus burden, and refractoriness to the endovascular treatment.

Key Points

- Thrombolytics remain an essential component of acute limb ischemia management
- Extended lysis using indwelling catheters markedly improves procedural success
- Delineation of distal target or runoff essential to planning treatment
- Rheolytic thrombectomy "power-pulse" mode best suited for same day intervention
- Distal embolic protection should be utilized when feasible to minimize risk of distal embolism

References

1 Hull, J.E., Hull, M.K., Urso, J.A., and Park, H.A. (2006). Tenecteplase in acute lower-leg ischemia: efficacy, dose, and adverse events. *J. Vasc. Interv. Radiol.* 17 (4): 629–636. https://doi.org/10.1097/01.RVI.0000202751.74625.79.

2 Castañeda, F., Swischuk, J.L., Li, R. et al. (2002). Declining-dose study of reteplase treatment for lower extremity arterial occlusions. *J. Vasc. Interv. Radiol.* 13 (11): 1093–1098. https://doi.org/10.1016/S1051-0443(07)61949-6.

3 Giannini, D. and Balbarini, A. (2005). Thrombolytic therapy in peripheral arterial disease. *Curr. Drug Target Cardiovas. Hematol. Disord.* 4 (3): 249–258. https://doi.org/10.2174/1568006043336113.

4 Morrison, H.L. (2006). Catheter-directed thrombolysis for acute limb ischemia. *Semin. Intervent. Radiol.* 23 (3): 258–269. https://doi.org/10.1055/s-2006-948765.

5 Semba, C.P., Matalon, T.A.S., Chopra, P. et al. (2000). Thrombolytic therapy with use of alteplase (rt-PA) in peripheral arterial occlusive disease: review of the clinical literature. *J. Vasc. Interv. Radiol.* 11 (2 I): 149–161. https://doi.org/10.1016/S1051-0443(07)61459-6.

6 Patel, N.II., Krishnamurthy, V.N., Kim, S. et al. (2013). Quality improvement guidelines for percutaneous management of acute lower-extremity ischemia. *J. Vasc. Interv. Radiol.* 24 (1): 3–15. https://doi.org/10.1016/j.jvir.2012.09.026.

7 Yusuf, S.W., Whitaker, S.C., Gregson, R.H.S. et al. (1995). Immediate and early follow-up results of pulse spray thrombolysis in patients with peripheral ischaemia. *Br. J. Surg.* 82 (3): 338–340. https://doi.org/10.1002/bjs.1800820318.

12

Pedal Reconstruction

Ehrin Armstrong and Rory Brinker

University of Colorado School of Medicine-Rocky Mountain Regional VA Medical Center, CO, USA

Introduction

An intact pedal arch is associated with improved wound healing in critical limb ischemia (CLI).

Endovascular treatment of the pedal arch has good procedural success and patient outcomes in published registries. The small vessel diameter and tortuous anatomy of the foot present unique challenges to endovascular intervention.

Pedal Arch Reconstruction

Arterial revascularization, by a surgical or endovascular approach, is recommended to prevent limb loss in critical limb ischemia (CLI) [1, 2]. Percutaneous transluminal angioplasty has been increasingly used in the treatment of infrainguinal arterial occlusive disease. While there are significant limitations in directly comparing endovascular and surgical first strategies for infrapopliteal occlusive disease in CLI, the limited data suggests comparable rates of limb salvage and survival, particularly in those with reduced life expectancy or without a suitable bypass vein graft [3–5].

A major goal of revascularization in CLI is to provide direct flow to the site of a nonhealing arterial wound. This can often necessitate multilevel intervention. Historically, most endovascular interventions were above the level of the ankle, but recent studies have suggested that inframalleolar intervention, including

Endovascular Interventions: A Step-by-Step Approach, First Edition. Edited by Jose M. Wiley, Cristina Sanina, George D. Dangas, and Prakash Krishnan.
© 2023 John Wiley & Sons Ltd. Published 2023 by John Wiley & Sons Ltd.

pedal arch angioplasty, may help improve wound healing rates. Therefore, the pedal arch is an important anatomic target in select CLI cases.

In the typical below knee anatomy, the popliteal artery gives rise to the anterior tibial (AT) artery and tibioperoneal trunk, which will in turn supply the peroneal and posterior tibial (PT) arteries. The peroneal artery will extend to the distal leg where it supplies the anterior malleolar and calcaneal branches. The AT courses to the forefoot where it transitions to the dorsalis pedis artery at the level of the ankle joint. The PT bifurcates below the malleolus into the medial and lateral plantar arteries (Figure 12.1), which in turn supply the plantar surface of the foot. Multiple anatomic variants of the below knee vasculature exist, including a trifurcating origin of the three vessels, high origins of the AT or PT, as well as hypoplasia of one or more branches. The absence of the PT is a more common variation, existing in 1–5% of the population [6].

The anterior circulation of the foot includes the dorsalis pedis, lateral tarsal, and arcuate arteries (Figure 12.2). The arcuate artery will typically supply the

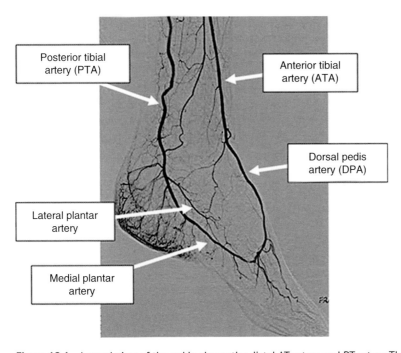

Figure 12.1 Lateral view of the ankle shows the distal AT artery and PT artery. The dorsalis pedis artery is a continuation of the AT artery. The PT artery bifurcates into the lateral plantar artery and medial plantar artery. *Source:* [6] Higashimori et al. (2017), Reproduced from IntechOpen.

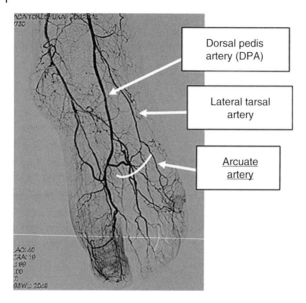

Figure 12.2 The anterior circulation consists of dorsalis pedis artery, lateral tarsal artery, and arcuate artery. *Source:* [6] Higashimori et al. (2017), Reproduced from IntechOpen.

second, third, and fourth dorsal metatarsal arteries, though anatomy is variable. The posterior foot circulation is composed of the medial and lateral plantar arteries, which connect via the deep plantar arch and give rise to the plantar metatarsal arteries (Figure 12.3) [6].

The pedal arch is the arterial connection between the anterior and posterior circulations of the foot in which the dorsalis pedis and lateral plantar arteries connect via the deep plantar. The pedal arch can have several anatomic variations which are clinically relevant to wound healing (Figure 12.4) [7, 8]. A complete pedal arch, as compared to interrupted pedal arch, has been associated with increased rates of wound healing and shorter time to healing in patients with CLI [9–11]. The presumed benefit of a complete pedal arch is the ability to collateralize adjacent angiosome territories resulting in the observed improvement in healing; however, the association of pedal arch quality and amputation-free survival for CLI has reported mixed results [10, 12].

Controlled investigations are needed to assess the association of anatomic pedal subtypes on clinical outcomes. While subject to publication bias, initial

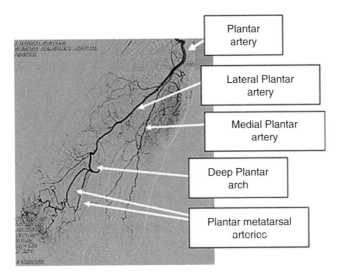

Figure 12.3 The posterior circulation consists of the medial plantar artery and lateral plantar artery. *Source:* [6] Higashimori et al. (2017), Reproduced from IntechOpen.

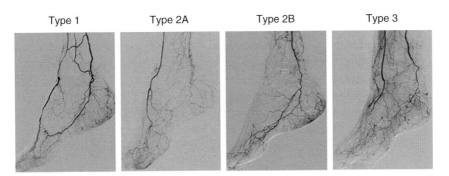

Figure 12.4 Pedal arch subtypes: Type 1: both dorsalis pedis and plantar arteries are patent; Type 2A: only dorsalis pedis artery is patent; B: only plantar artery patent; 3: both dorsalis pedis and plantar arteries are occluded. *Source:* [7] Kawarada et al. (2012), Reproduced from John Wiley & Sons.

observational series of pedal arch intervention have been promising. In single center and multicenter registries, endovascular angioplasty of the transpedal arch has resulted in favorable outcomes, with technical success rates of 75–88% [9, 11, 13], limb salvage rate of 88%, and amputation-free survival rate of 73% at one year [9]. When care is taken to avoid injury to a potential infrapopliteal surgical target vessel, an endovascular first approach has not shown negative impact to surgical pedal bypass outcomes [14].

Endovascular intervention of the pedal arch has been shown to be a safe and effective approach to treatment and has become an important intervention target in select CLI cases. This chapter will focus on the unique challenges and a systematic approach to pedal arch intervention.

Indications for Pedal Revascularization

Current guidelines do not differentiate pedal from infrapopliteal revascularization recommendations in the setting of CLI. The goals of transpedal arch intervention are to improve outflow of the tibial arteries, to improve flow to an adjacent angiosome, and to open a conduit for retrograde intervention of an additional infratibial vessel to achieve in-line flow in CLI. Procedural failure may result in worsening foot ischemia, so appropriate patient selection is crucial. When care is taken to avoid injury to a potential surgical target vessel, an endovascular first approach has shown to not have a negative impact on surgical pedal bypass outcomes (Figures 12.5 a–h and 12.6a–d) [14].

Technical Considerations

Pedal arch intervention is best approached via the ipsilateral antegrade approach. The pedal vessels are small in caliber and take a more tortuous course than the larger and more proximal leg vessels. An antegrade approach with a long sheath maximizes the ability to push and transmit torque for wire and catheter manipulation. A long sheath will also allow the use of shorter length catheters, devices, and wires, which can become a significant limitation of alternative access strategies. Placing the sheath in the most distal disease-free segment of the superficial femoral artery (SFA) can maximize support. A 5 Fr system will enable passage of equipment needed for the small caliber infratibial and pedal vessels, though if there are plans to use a closure device that requires a larger arteriotomy, a 6 Fr system is also commonly used.

Access

1) Obtain antegrade ipsilateral common femoral artery access via modified Seldinger technique under direct ultrasound guidance utilizing a micropuncture access kit.

2) Place a 5 or 6 Fr × 23 cm length or longer sheath over a 0.035 stiff wire with soft tip (Hi-Torque Supra Core – Abbott, Santa Clara, CA, USA). Advance the sheath tip to the most distal nondiseased SFA vessel segment.
3) After sheath placement, administer unfractionated heparin with a goal activated clotting time (ACT) of 250–300 seconds.

Lesion Crossing

Non-chronic total occlusion (CTO) Lesion Subtype:

1) For non-CTO lesions, a workhorse wire can be used, though given the small caliber and tortuosity, often a hydrophilic or polymer jacketed 0.014 tapered wire such as a Fielder XT (Abbott, Santa Clara, CA, USA) is required to navigate the distal vessels.
2) A 0.014 microcatheter may be required for crossing support (Corsair–Asahi Intecc, Irvine, CA, USA), CXI (Cook, Bloomington, IN, USA), Quick-cross (Philips, San Diego, CA, USA), Turnpike LP (Teleflex, Morrisville, NC, USA).

CTO Lesion Subtype

– See chapter on CTO crossing for technique. Techniques used for lesion crossing in the distal infratibial and pedal vessels are similar to those used for coronary CTO intervention.
– Subintimal crossing should be approached with caution as extension of a subintimal plane can occlude branch vessels of the arch with potential worsening perfusion that can lead to tissue or limb loss. True lumen crossing is essential for maximizing tissue perfusion.

Special Considerations of the Pedal Intervention

Defining Pedal Anatomy: Selective angiography via long sheath or through a microcatheter (e.g. 0.035 Navicross – Terumo, or 0.018 Quick-cross – Spectranetics) is recommended to deliver concentrated contrast injections to the infrapopliteal and pedal vessels for optimal anatomic definition prior to and during intervention. Standard views include AP with shallow cranial and straight lateral views of the foot.

Lumen Crossing: Due to the branch and choke vessels that arise from the pedal arch, subintimal crossing and recanalization can lead to branch occlusion with the risk of tissue or limb loss. Every effort should be made to cross true lumen.

Anticoagulation Strategy: Given small caliber vessels with diminished flow, anticoagulation levels must be judiciously watched with a goal ACT between 250 and 300 seconds to avoid thrombus formation.

Vessel Tortuosity: Tortuosity can be a challenge in small vessels. Difficult to cross lesions may be better defined by taking additional, nonstandard oblique angiographic views for better spatial understanding and directionality of the vessel. In addition, plantar or dorsiflexion of the foot may enable changes in vessel conformation to allow wire or device passage through tortuosity near the ankle [7].

Vasospasm: Small caliber vessels are more prone to vasospasm. Liberal use of intraarterial vasodilators is recommended. Verapamil dosed at 2.5 mg and nitroglycerin dosed at 200 mcg are commonly used and will be most effective when delivered via a microcatheter.

Angioplasty Technique and Balloon Sizing: Bailout stenting below the ankle is not recommended, so care should be taken to achieve optimal angioplasty result. Low pressure, prolonged inflations (e.g. three minutes), and 1 : 1 balloon sizing are recommended. Infrapopliteal vessel sizing can be accomplished using an IVUS catheter if vessel caliber allows. In practice, tortuosity and small vessel caliber prevent the use of intravascular imaging for vessels below the ankle. Most infrapopliteal vessels will measure 1.5–2.5 mm. A 1.5–2.0 mm balloon is most commonly used for the dorsalis pedis, pedal arch, and plantar arteries. Angiography following administration of vasodilators through a microcatheter can aid in estimation of vessel caliber. When there is question of sizing, the smaller of balloons should be chosen to minimize risk of flow limiting dissection or perforation.

Calcification: Calcification of the pedal arch vessels poses a challenge, particularly in tortuous vessels. The pedal arch vessels are not large enough to accommodate scoring balloons. In straight vessel segments, orbital atherectomy can be performed using a 1.25 mm micro crown (Cardiovascular Systems, Inc). Due to short anatomic landing zone and small caliber vessels, distal embolic filter protection is not possible. Similar to coronary intervention, atherectomy runs must be limited in duration, ideally less than 10 seconds, to allow for adequate washout to prevent the no-reflow phenomenon. Tortuosity increases the risk of vessel dissection or perforation during atherectomy. In such cases, a small coronary balloon can be utilized for focal angioplasty at higher pressure if required for a recalcitrant calcified lesion. Ultimately, calcification with tortuosity increases the risk of the procedure and the operator should reassess the risk and benefit of proceeding.

Troubleshooting

Uncrossable Lesion: Standard CTO crossing techniques including wire escalation can also be employed in the foot. Subintimal crossing and reentry in these small vessels is not recommended as this may result in occlusion of branch vessels, and stenting in the foot for bailout is not recommended.

Inability to Deliver a Catheter or Balloon: When confronted with complex infrapopliteal and pedal arch lesions, it is important to maximize access and sheath support during preprocedural planning as described previously. Next, use a low-profile balloon such as a 1.5 mm Advance LP (Cook Medical) or 1.0 mm Sapphire (Cardiovascular Systems Incorporated). If the uncrossable lesion is at the level of the ankle, attempt a different flexion, extension, or rotation of the foot to change the geometric relationship between the balloon, wire, and vessel. Using stiffer wires (e.g. Viper and Wiggle) can also be effective, though the use of these are associated with an increased risk of small vessel perforation and this risk should be factored into the decision to escalate.

Diffuse Small Vessel Disease: "Desert Foot" is a challenging scenario in which there is minimal global perfusion of the foot due to diffuse severe small vessel disease. This entity is generally not amenable to endovascular intervention, although in select cases it may be possible to reconstruct the pedal loop if the inflow vessels are of sufficient diameter.

Vessel Perforation: Perforation or severe dissection of a small vessel in the foot should be controlled by prolonged balloon inflation. Placing a coronary stent to the foot is not recommended, given the flexion forces and high risk for stent disruption and thrombosis. Perforation of the below ankle vessels can typically be managed by external manual compression. The limited number of bailout strategies available and risk of vessel closure in treating these complications should be considered in the initial risk/benefit determination as to whether the patient may benefit from intervention.

Summary

The quality of the pedal arch is an important predictor of wound healing in CLI. Advances in endovascular technique have allowed endovascular intervention of the pedal arch to achieve good efficacy and safety outcomes. With appropriate patient selection and technique, the pedal arch can be a valuable intervention target in CLI.

Case Example 1

A 65-year-old male with 5×5 cm left heel ulceration with black eschar, concern for early osteomyelitis, and a toe pressure of 12 mmHg (Wifi score: three infections, two to three wound, one infection) (Figure 12.5a–h).

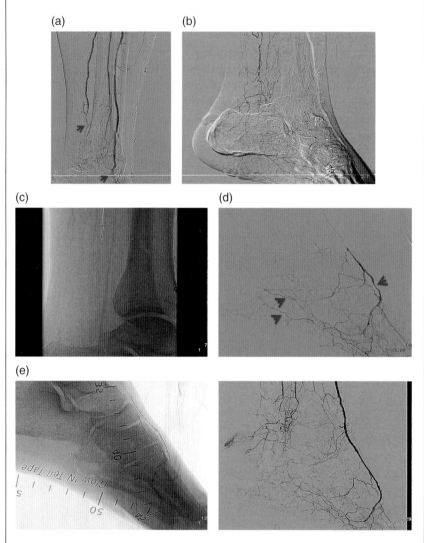

Figure 12.5 (a) Occlusion of distal PT artery and severe stenosis of distal dorsalis pedis artery. (b) Lateral view demonstrating poor heel wound perfusion. (c) The distal PT artery is severely calcified and was unable to be crossed antegrade with a wire escalation strategy using an Astato 30 (ASAHI INTECC CO., LTD.). (d) Severe stenosis of the distal dorsalis pedis with intact pedal arch supplying the medial and lateral plantar arches. (e) The pedal arch was successfully crossed with a hydrophilic Fielder XT wire (Abbott). (f) Orbital atherectomy was performed using a 1.25 mm crown CSI catheter. (g) Prolonged balloon angioplasty was performed across the pedal arch with a 2.0 mm Advance LP (Cook Medical) balloon. (h) Final angiography demonstrating improved perfusion through the arch into the plantar branches.

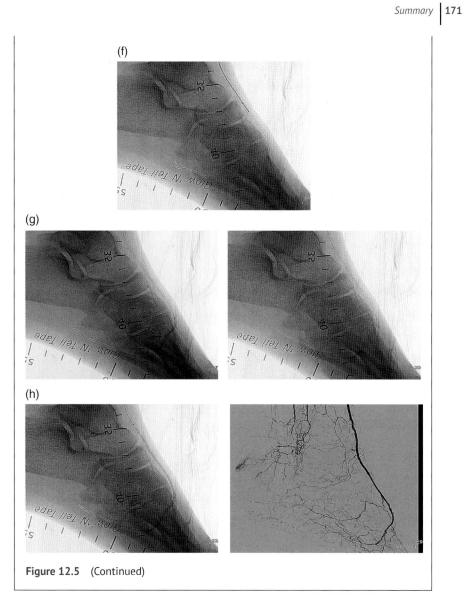

(f)

(g)

(h)

Figure 12.5 (Continued)

Case Example 2

A 67-year-old male with CLI and nonhealing wound of the right hallux. Angiography demonstrated a densely calcified long segment occlusion of the proximal AT with unsuccessful wiring via the antegrade approach (Figure 12.6a–d).

(a)   (b)

(c)   (d)

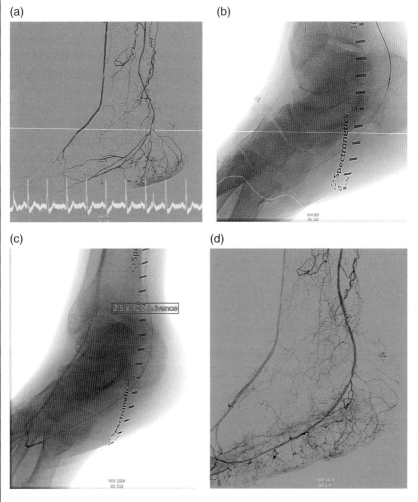

Figure 12.6   (a) Severe stenoses of the distal AT, distal PT, and dorsalis pedis with an uninterrupted pedal arch. (b) The PT stenosis and pedal arch was wired using Runthrough wire (Terumo) and corsair microcatheter for support. (c) Prolonged balloon angioplasty was performed with 2.5 mm Advance LP balloon (Cook Medical). (d) Final angiography demonstrating improved perfusion in the PT, pedal arch, and dorsalis pedis. The intervention enabled a retrograde approach to the proximal AT CTO.

References

1 Norgren, L., Hiatt, W.R., Dormandy, J.A. et al. (2007). Inter-society consensus for the management of peripheral arterial disease (TASC II). *Eur. J. Vasc. Endovasc. Surg.* 33 (1): https://doi.org/10.1016/j.ejvs.2006.09.024.

2 Gerhard-Herman, M.D., Gornik, H.L., Barrett, C. et al. (2017). 2016 AHA/ACC Guideline on the management of patients with lower extremity peripheral artery disease: a report of the American College of Cardiology/American Heart Association Task Force on Clinical Practice Guidelines [published correction appears in Circulation. 2017 Mar 21;135(12):e791–e792]. *Circulation* 135 (12): e726–e779. https://doi.org/10.1161/CIR.0000000000000471.

3 Romiti, M., Albers, M., Brochado-Neto, F.C. et al. (2008). Meta-analysis of infrapopliteal angioplasty for chronic critical limb ischemia. *J. Vasc. Surg.* 47: 975–981.

4 Bradbury, A.W., Adam, D.J., Bell, J. et al. (2010). Bypass versus Angioplasty in Severe Ischaemia of the Leg (BASIL) trial: an intention-to-treat analysis of amputation-free and overall survival in patients randomized to a bypass surgery-first or a balloon angioplasty-first revascularization strategy. *J. Vasc. Surg.* 51 (5): https://doi.org/10.1016/j.jvs.2010.01.073.

5 Almasri, J., Adusumalli, J., Asi, N. et al. (2019). A systematic review and meta-analysis of revascularization outcomes of infrainguinal chronic limb-threatening ischemia. *J. Vasc. Surg.* 69 (6): https://doi.org/10.1016/j.jvs.2018.01.071.

6 Higashimori, A. (2017). *Angiography and Endovascular Therapy for Below-the-Knee Artery Disease, Angiography and Endovascular Therapy for Peripheral Artery Disease* (ed. Y. Yokoi, K. Fukuda, M. Fujihara, et al.). IntechOpen https://doi.org/10.5772/67179.

7 Kawarada, O., Fujihara, M., Higashimori, A. et al. (2012). Predictors of adverse clinical outcomes after successful infrapopliteal intervention. *Catheter. Cardiovasc. Interv.* 80 (5): 861–871. https://doi.org/10.1002/ccd.24370.

8 Kawarada, O., Sakamoto, S., Harada, K. et al. (2014). Contemporary crossing techniques for infrapopliteal chronic Total occlusions. *J. Endovasc. Ther.* 21 (2): 266–280. https://doi.org/10.1583/13-4460mr.1.

9 Nakama, T., Watanabe, N., Haraguchi, T. et al. (2017). TCTAP A-124 clinical outcomes of pedal artery angioplasty for patients with ischemic wounds; results from the multicenter rendezvous registry. *J. Am. Coll. Cardiol.* 69: –16. https://doi.org/10.1016/j.jacc.2017.03.167.

10 Rashid, H., Slim, H., Zayed, H. et al. (2013). The impact of arterial pedal arch quality and angiosome revascularization on foot tissue loss healing and infrapopliteal bypass outcome. *J. Vasc. Surg.* 57: 1219–1226.

11 Cheun, T.J., Jayakumar, L., Sideman, M.J. et al. (2020). Outcomes of isolated inframalleolar interventions for chronic limb-threatening ischemia in diabetic patients. *J. Vasc. Surg.* 71 (5): 1644–1652.e2. https://doi.org/10.1016/j.jvs.2019.07.094.

12 Higashimori, A., Iida, O., Yamauchi, Y. et al. (2015). Outcomes of one straight-line flow with and without pedal arch in patients with critical limb ischemia. *Catheter. Cardiovasc. Interv.* 87 (1): 129–133. https://doi.org/10.1002/ccd.26164.

13 Graziani, L. (2017). Crossing the Rubicon: a closer look at the pedal loop technique. *Ann. Vasc. Surg.* 45: 315–323. https://doi.org/10.1016/j.avsg.2017.06.135.

14 Uhl, C., Hock, C., Betz, T. et al. (2014). Pedal bypass surgery after Crural endovascular intervention. *J. Vasc. Surg.* 59 (6): 1583–1587. https://doi.org/10.1016/j.jvs.2013.11.071.

13

Endovascular Management of Access Site Complications

Manaf Assafin[1], Robert Pyo[2], Pedro Cox-Alomar[3], and Miguel Alvarez-Villela[1]

[1] *Division of Cardiology, Albert Einstein College of Medicine-Montefiore Medical Center, Bronx, NY, USA*
[2] *Division of Cardiology, Renaissance School of Medicine at Stony Brook University, NY, USA*
[3] *Division of Cardiology, Louisiana State University School of Medicine, New Orleans, LA, USA*

Introduction

Percutaneous endovascular procedures always begin and end with the vascular access. Unfortunately, complications related to the access site are relatively common and result in additional morbidity to patients and increased costs to health systems. In the modern era of increasing procedure complexity, it is imperative for the interventional physician to be aware of these complications and understand the basic techniques to treat or mitigate them. In this chapter, we review the most common complications associated with vascular access, describe a variety of endovascular management options, and discuss the indications for escalation to surgical management.Arterial access site complications are common after cardiac or endovascular catheterization, with the incidence related to procedure complexity and vascular access bore size [1, 2], and has been cited as ranging from 1.8% for diagnostic procedures to 9% for interventional procedures [3]. Recent improvements in procedural technique and device technology, as well as the increasing utilization of mechanical support devices, have led to an increase in procedure complexity and large bore vascular access. It is therefore prudent for the practicing interventional operator to be familiar with vascular complications and their management.

Endovascular Interventions: A Step-by-Step Approach, First Edition. Edited by Jose M. Wiley, Cristina Sanina, George D. Dangas, and Prakash Krishnan.
© 2023 John Wiley & Sons Ltd. Published 2023 by John Wiley & Sons Ltd.

Table 13.1 Common arterial access complications by access site.

Femoral artery	Radial artery
Retroperitoneal Hematoma	Radial artery spasm
Femoral Artery Pseudoaneurysm (FAP)	Radial artery occlusion
Arteriovenous fistula formation	Hematoma formation
Femoral Artery Occlusion	Radial artery perforation

This chapter will focus on the practical management of common access site complications after percutaneous coronary or endovascular interventions. A list of common complications sorted by arterial access site is provided in Table 13.1.

Complications Related to Common Femoral Artery Access

The most common femoral artery (CFA) related complications include local bleeding, retroperitoneal hematomas (RPH), femoral artery pseudoaneurysms (PSA), arteriovenous fistulae (AVF), and lower extremity ischemia due to thrombosis or embolization. Although surgical treatment may be possible in nearly all cases of femoral injury, surgery has been associated with a 25% postoperative morbidity and 3.5% postoperative mortality in some series, a risk that reflects the highly comorbid profile of this subset of patients [4], while endovascular techniques have in most cases become the primary approach to the management of these complications. Table 13.2 lists some of the most common femoral arterial complications and their management options.

Access Site Bleeding

Access site bleeding in patients undergoing percutaneous coronary intervention (PCI) is the most common periprocedural complication (2–12%). Several studies have found major bleeding after PCI to be an independent predictor of mortality [5–7].

Risk factors for access site bleeding can be categorized into patient-related and procedure-related factors (Table 13.3). Patient-related factors which increase this risk include female gender, age > 70 years, a small body surface area (<1.6 m^2), history of heart failure, chronic obstructive pulmonary disease (COPD), peripheral vascular disease, triple vessel coronary artery disease, concomitant shock,

Table 13.2 Most common femoral arterial complications and their management options.

Complication type	Overall incidence after percutaneous coronary intervention (PCI)	Treatment options
Retroperitoneal hematoma	0.4–0.74%	• Hemostasis by prolonged balloon inflation over extravasation site • Covered stent placement • Surgery for rare selected cases
Femoral artery pseudoaneurysm (FAP)	2–6%	• Ultrasound-guided compression repair • Percutaneous thrombin injection • Biodegradable collagen injection • Covered stent placement • Coil embolization • Surgery reserved for very large aneurysms
Arteriovenous fistula formation	0.4%	• Conservative in asymptomatic patients • Ultrasound-guided compression repair • Arterial covered stent placement in symptomatic patients
Femoral artery occlusion	<0.5%	• Balloon angioplasty • Catheter-directed thrombolysis • Catheter thrombectomy • Covered stent placement • Surgery for endovascular treatment failure

and renal failure (sCr > 2 mg/dl) [8, 9]. Procedure-related factors include large arterial sheath size (7–8 Fr vs. 6 Fr, 23.5% vs. 13.8%; p < 0.01), [2] prolonged heparin infusion after PCI [10], delayed sheath removal [11], emergent procedures, and periprocedural use of GP IIb/IIIa inhibitors [9, 11], especially when concomitant heparin administration leads to supratherapeutic clotting times [8, 12].

Management of access site bleeding is dictated by its site, severity, and hemodynamic consequences. In most cases, localized femoral bleeding and hematomas

Table 13.3 Risk factors for bleeding complications after femoral arterial access.

Risk factors for bleeding related to femoral artery access
Female gender
Age > 70 yr
Body surface area < 1.6 m^2
Renal failure with a serum Cr > 2 mg/dl
Prolonged indwelling sheath time
Larger sheath diameter
Emergent procedures
Larger heparin dose and prolonged heparin infusion
Use of GP IIb/IIIa inhibitors

can be controlled with local manual or mechanical compression, discontinuation of anticoagulants, and in some cases reversal of therapeutic anticoagulation.

In the case of GP IIb/IIIa inhibitors, reversal of anticoagulation requires special considerations. Reversal can be achieved with platelet transfusions when abciximab (ReoPro, Eli Lilly, Indianapolis, IN, USA) has been used, as this agent binds tightly to circulating platelets but will not affect the activity of normally functioning transfused platelets. Small molecule platelet GP IIb/IIIa inhibitors like eptifibatide (Integrilin, Cor Therapeutics, South San Francisco, CA, USA) and tirofiban (Aggrastat, Merck, West Point, PA, USA) may be harder to reverse with transfusion since they act as competitive, reversible receptor inhibitors and leave excess free circulating drug that may affect newly transfused platelets. However, their shorter half-life will allow for the antiplatelet effect to cease after about 4 hours compared to 12 hours with abciximab.

Retroperitoneal hematoma or hemorrhage (RPH) is arguably the most grave access site bleeding complication. It has an incidence of 0.4–0.74% after PCI and is associated with significant morbidity and mortality. Besides the known risk factors for bleeding, a puncture of the CFA above the middle third of the femoral head, insertion of the sheath above the inguinal ligament, and punctures of the back wall are associated with increased risk of RPH.

It is important to note that RPH remains a clinical diagnosis and requires a high index of suspicion. Early symptoms are nonspecific and include back pain, groin pain, or ipsilateral lower quadrant abdominal tenderness, followed by relative hypotension, tachycardia, and hypovolemic shock. The majority of patients with RPH present within three hours of the index procedure; therefore, patients presenting in this window with hypotension should be promptly evaluated for RPH [13–15].

In cases where bleeding is more severe or uncompressible, swift endovascular management is prudent. One of the most fundamental endovascular skills for management of femoral arterial access site complications is the "up and over" or "crossover" technique, which is the mainstay for most endovascular interventions performed on the femoral artery from the contralateral side. This will be briefly reviewed here.

Crossover Technique

Step 1. The contralateral CFA is cannulated over the femoral head using fluoroscopic and ultrasound (US) guidance, 1–2 cm above the femoral bifurcation and below the origin of the inferior epigastric artery.

Step 2. A 5 Fr diagnostic internal mammary (IMA) or Omni Flush (Angiodynamics, Latham, NY, USA) catheter is advanced over a steerable 0.035″ wire with a floppy tip – such as a Wholey (Medtronic, Dublin, Ireland) into the thoracic descending aorta.

Step 3. The steerable wire is pulled back into the catheter, which is then gently torqued and withdrawn until its tip engages the ostium of the contralateral common iliac artery. This can be confirmed by advancing the Wholey wire beyond the tip of the catheter and observing its course before removing it from the body.

Step 4. After confirming normal arterial waveform, digital subtraction angiography (DSA) of the contralateral iliofemoral system is performed with the image intensifier angulated approximately 30° contralateral to the side of interest.

Step 5. Once the area of bleeding is identified, the wire is again advanced through the iliofemoral system into the superficial femoral artery (SFA) or the profunda artery. The diagnostic catheter is then removed, and the short femoral sheath is replaced with a long 6 Fr sheath over the wire, with the tip positioned proximal to the area of interest.

Retrograde access via the "up and over" technique forms the basis for most strategies for endovascular management of access site complications.

Balloon Tamponade, Endovascular Coiling, and Covered Stent Placement

In the case of access site bleeding, balloon tamponade is often sufficient to achieve hemostasis. With a wire across the area of bleeding and a long sheath tip proximal to the area of interest, a peripheral balloon sized 1 : 1 to the vessel is advanced to the area of bleeding and inflated at 6–8 atm in five-minute intervals, followed by brief (30-second) periods with the balloon deflated to allow for antegrade flow and assess hemostasis. Complete occlusion of the vessel should be confirmed by DSA from the contralateral sheath.

If there is persistent bleeding after prolonged balloon tamponade, one must consider the site of bleeding to determine the appropriate next step. Bleeding involving very distal or small branch vessels may be appropriate to treat with coil embolization. This is achieved by advancing a guide catheter of appropriate shape (e.g. a multipurpose, Judkins right, or IMA catheter) to the vessel of interest, and then advancing a wire followed by a microcatheter into the vessel. The wire is then retracted, and 0.014″ or 0.018″ coils are then advanced through the microcatheter and delivered tightly into the bleeding vessel. If the bleeding vessel is collateralized, coils should be delivered both proximal and distal to the area of bleeding in order to prevent retrograde flow and continued bleeding (Figure 13.1a–d).

Bleeding involving larger vessels not responding to balloon occlusion should prompt consideration of a covered stent-graft placement. After appropriate anticoagulation is administered, a covered stent with a diameter 1 mm larger than the native vessel should be advanced under fluoroscopy from the contralateral sheath, with enough proximal and distal landing zones to ensure adequate sealing. However, careful attention should be paid to avoid crossing the CFA bifurcation in order to prevent obstruction of the ostia of the deep femoral artery (DFA) or SFA. Self-expanding nitinol-framed stent-grafts are preferred in areas such as the hip joint near the flexion point of the inguinal ligament, as they have been shown to have increased fatigue resistance to bending, crushing, and stretching [16]; however, their longer lengths and less precise deployment can make their use challenging. Balloon-expandable stent-grafts are available in shorter lengths and can be more precisely deployed; however, stent deformation is a concern when they are used near flexion points.

A completion angiogram should always be performed to ensure there is cessation of bleeding and patency of the SFA and DFA, keeping in mind that postdilation of the stent-graft may be necessary if there is continued extravasation. In cases where covered stent-graft placement is unsuccessful, or not feasible due to anatomy (tortuous/calcified iliac arteries, or bleeding directly at the bifurcation of the CFA), surgical consultation for open repair should be pursued.

Femoral Pseudoaneurysms

A femoral PSA forms when a breach of all three layers of the arterial wall results in a hematoma that remains in continued communication with the arterial lumen. Similar to a hematoma, the hemorrhage and resulting blood collection is contained by the adventitia or perivascular soft tissue; but unlike a hematoma, there is continued flow of blood into the PSA sac in systole and out of the sac in diastole.

(a)

(b)

(c)

(d)

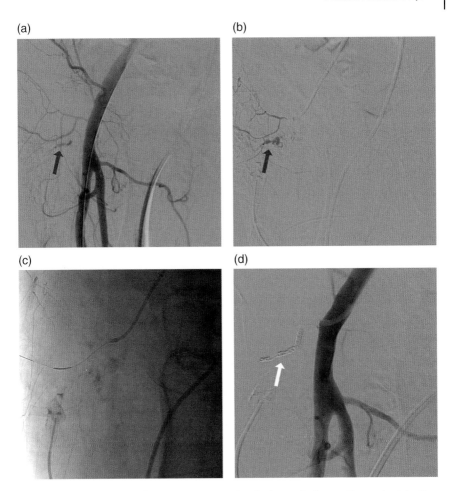

Figure 13.1 Bleeding and contrast extravasation (red arrow) of a small vessel originating from the CFA after cardiac catheterization (a). Selective cannulation and angiography of the vessel with a Judkins right catheter from the contralateral femoral artery (b), followed by advancement of a coronary wire and microcatheter (c), and finally 0.14″ coil placement (Axium detachable coils, Medtronic) (white arrows) (d) with final angiography showing no residual bleeding.

The reported incidence of femoral PSA ranges from 2% to 6% after peripheral or coronary interventions, and less than 0.5% after diagnostic angiography [17, 18]. Larger bore access, more aggressive anticoagulant and antiplatelet therapy use, simultaneous ipsilateral femoral vein and artery catheterization, and lower punctures, especially when they result in SFA cannulation, are all associated with increased risk of PSA formation [19]. PSAs are also more common in women, patients over the age of 70 years, diabetics, and those with obesity [20].

Clinically, femoral PSAs present with pain, swelling, and bruising at the site of a recent arterial puncture, and examination often reveals a palpable thrill or pulsatile mass. The gravest complication related to femoral PSAs is rupture, but other complications include persistent local pain, infection, embolization of thrombus from the PSA to the distal circulation, or issues resulting from compression of adjacent structures (e.g. femoral nerve palsy with femoral nerve compression, or deep venous thrombosis [DVT] with femoral vein compression).

Duplex US is the preferred modality for diagnosis and serial evaluation of arterial PSA. The study should seek to identify the site of origin of the aneurysm from the parent vessel, the waveform pattern of the inflow and outflow arterial tree, the size of the aneurysm including the number of loculations, and the length and diameter of the aneurysm neck. These anatomic features are crucial in dictating the appropriate treatment strategy.

Although there is some discrepancy in the published literature regarding the threshold to undergo treatment, it is generally accepted that femoral PSAs less than 2 cm in diameter are excepted to resolve spontaneously and could be reasonably managed conservatively, though close follow-up with serial arterial duplex US should be performed to confirm resolution.

PSAs larger than 2 cm generally require treatment. Although traditionally treated surgically, minimally invasive techniques have become the initial treatment strategy since 1991 when Fellmeth and colleagues introduced a minimally invasive approach to thrombose iatrogenic PSAs by externally compressing the PSA with US guidance, with a success rate of 93% [21]. Ultrasound-guided compression repair (UGCR) has become a widely adopted initial strategy in stable patients with simple femoral PSAs. Modern series report technical success rates between 75% and 98% [22–25]; however, in patients on anticoagulation a failure rate as high as 30–40% has been documented [26].

Ultrasound-Guided Compression Repair

Step 1. Using a 5 or 7 MHz linear or curvilinear probe, the neck of the PSA is identified using color flow Doppler.

Step 2. Manual compression is applied to the neck via the transducer, in order to prevent flow into the PSA sac on color Doppler.

Step 3. Continuous pressure is applied while monitoring flow into the aneurysm sac for approximately 10 minutes.

Step 4. Pressure is slowly released and flow into the PSA sac is assessed (see Figure 13.2a,b).

The steps are repeated until either the patient can no longer tolerate the discomfort, the operator can no longer continue due to fatigue, or the PSA thromboses.

(a) (b)

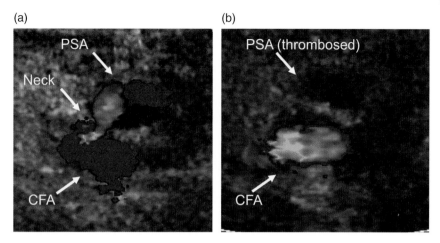

Figure 13.2 Pseudoaneurysm arising from the CFA as demonstrated by color duplex ultrasonography (a). Successful thrombosis of PSA after UGCR with cessation of flow into the PSA sac (b).

Compression times of up to 300 minutes can be required, though the average compression time is about 30 minutes. Analgesia and/or sedation may be required for the patient to tolerate the procedure. Although effective and noninvasive, patient discomfort and significant labor/time intensiveness have limited this technique's widespread adoption in the modern era.

Ultrasound-Guided Thrombin Injection

An increasingly attractive option to treat PSA is the US-guided injection of thrombin to elicit thrombosis of the aneurysm sac. Technical ease, minimal patient discomfort, and high procedural success rates have made this the favored primary approach for the treatment of PSAs in many institutions, including ours. The procedure can be safely performed at the bedside or in the catheterization laboratory, and requires only an assistant and standard US equipment and needles. Technical success rates are high, and have been reported in the range of 90–100% [27–30]. We prefer human thrombin as opposed to bovine in order to minimize the risk of allergic reaction.

Step 1. 1000 IU human thrombin in 1 ml of normal saline is suspended to yield a concentration of 1000 IU/ml.

Step 2. A three-way stopcock is prepared with an appropriate needle (most PSAs can be treated with a 1.5 in. 22-gauge needle), and two 1 cc syringes, one with thrombin and the other with normal saline.

Step 3. Under US guidance, the tip of the needle is slowly advanced into the PSA sac, directed toward the base of the sac and away from the neck of the PSA.

Step 4. Ensuring the saline syringe is "on" and the thrombin syringe is "off" on the three-way stopcock, 5 ml of saline are injected while monitoring the color Doppler signal to ensure the tip of the needle is in the desired location.

Step 5. After satisfactory position is confirmed, the three-way stopcock is turned so the thrombin syringe is "on" and 300 IU (0.3 ml) of thrombin are injected into the PSA sac.

Step 6. Monitor for thrombus formation and cessation flow in the PSA. If flow remains after 10 minutes, repeat the process as needed.

Most PSAs can be thrombosed with 1000 IU thrombin, but rarely more may be required. Bed rest is generally advised for 6–12 hours after the procedure. A repeat duplex US should be performed 24 hours after thrombin injection, and again in one to two weeks to ensure resolution of the PSA.

Embolization of thrombin into the native arterial tree is a rare but real complication of this method, and may result in distal thrombosis which may require emergent angiography using contralateral retrograde femoral access, mechanical thrombectomy, and/or intraarterial thrombolysis. In PSAs with absent or short, wide necks (>5 mm), balloon occlusion of the parent vessel over the mouth of the PSA during thrombin injection has been suggested as a way to reduce the risk for thrombin embolization; however, data is lacking to support this.

Covered Stent Placement

Covered stent placement may be used to exclude PSAs from the circulation in cases not treatable by percutaneous compression of thrombin injection, and can be a good alternative to surgery. For example, PSAs of the SFA or DFA can be treated with short covered stents to avoid crossing into the CFA, maintaining a site for possible future catheterization while preserving vessel patency. Several small series have reported a high success rate in treating PSAs using covered stents [31, 32]. As previously mentioned, care must be taken to avoid deploying covered stent-grafts near the CFA bifurcation in order to avoid occlusion of the SFA or DFA. Covered stent-grafts should be used judiciously in younger patients, as long-term patency remains a concern [32].

Other Techniques

Other percutaneous techniques for the treatment of PSAs include transarterial thrombin injection, coil embolization, and percutaneous collagen injection. Transarterial thrombin injection may allow thrombin delivery to sites not

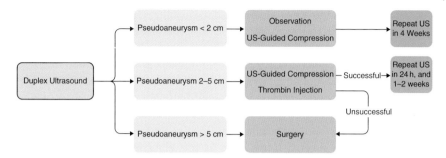

Figure 13.3 Algorithm for the management of femoral pseudoaneurysms.

otherwise accessible percutaneously, such as the DFA, but requires contralateral arterial access. Coil embolization, either percutaneous or transarterial, leads to thrombosis of the PSA; however, it also risks increasing PSA pressure possibly leading to rupture, as well as preventing shrinkage of the PSA after occlusion, and may act as a nidus for infection [33]. The percutaneous injection of a collagen paste or plug is an alternative to percutaneous thrombin injection; however, it requires a larger needle or even sheath for delivery, and is generally not favored compared to thrombin.

Surgical treatment of PSAs should be considered in very large (>5 cm) or rapidly expanding PSAs, symptoms associated with local compression (neuropathy, local ischemic changes, etc.), an infected PSA, or failure of percutaneous therapies. An algorithm for the management of femoral PSA is described in Figure 13.3.

Arteriovenous Fistulas

An arteriovenous fistula (AVF) refers to an abnormal communication between an adjacent artery and vein. This can occur when an access needle and introducer sheath are inserted through both vessels, thus allowing for shunting from artery to vein upon sheath removal. The incidence of femoral AVF after cardiac catheterization has been cited to be less than <1% [34, 35]. Factors associated with femoral AVF formation include a low puncture (below the bifurcation of the CFA), multiple puncture attempts, ipsilateral arterial and venous cannulation, and prolonged clotting times during the procedure [20].

Clinically, most patients with AVFs are asymptomatic, and the shunt is usually discovered incidentally after clinical examination reveals a palpable thrill and a "to and fro" murmur on auscultation. The presence of classical examination findings should prompt duplex ultrasonography which confirms the diagnosis. Most AVFs are of no significant clinical consequence and will close spontaneously.

Uncommonly, high output heart failure, arterial insufficiency, or venous congestive symptoms may occur. In these rare instances, percutaneous or surgical closure is indicated.

Some cases may respond to US-guided compression; however commonly, these patients are on antithrombotic therapy for comorbid cardiovascular disease, and have AVFs in less compressible areas below the femoral head, both of which decrease the efficacy of this technique. Covered stent placement on the arterial side of the AVF has been associated with high success and patency rates [31]. Balloon-expandable covered stents such as the Viabahn VBX (Gore Medical, Flagstaff, AZ, USA) allow for precise placement and are available in shorter lengths than their self-expanding counterparts, making them ideal for this application, especially in AVFs of the SFA and DFA where stent deformation is of lower concern. Surgical referral is indicated in cases where less invasive techniques fail or are not feasible.

Vascular Closure Device Related Complications

Vascular closure devices (VCD), first developed in the mid-1990s, have been a novel means to improve patient comfort and allow for early ambulation after endovascular procedures performed from the femoral artery. VCDs may be categorized based on their mechanism of action: active closure devices include suture-mediated devices (Perclose, Abbott Vascular, Redwood City, CA, USA), bioresorbable intravascular anchor/extravascular collagen implant (Angioseal, Terumo Medical, Somerset, NJ, USA; MANTA, Teleflex, Morrisville, NC, USA), and surgical staple/clip technology (Starclose, Abbot Vascular, Redwood City, CA, USA). Passive VCDs are a heterogenous group that is often used in conjunction with manual compression to achieve hemostasis, and include procoagulant patches, compression devices, and soluble extravascular sealants (Mynx, Cordis, Santa Clara, CA, USA). A list of the most common VCDs, their mechanism, and sheath sizes is detailed in Table 13.4.

The most common complications associated with VCD use include bleeding due to device failure, infection, and acute vessel closure; the last of which requires the most urgent recognition and treatment to prevent ischemic complications.

Suture-mediated or collagen plug VCDs have an intravascular component which can lead to vascular stenosis or occlusion by various mechanisms, including suturing of the posterior femoral arterial wall [36]. In the case of collagen plug devices, vessel closure can occur by interaction of the intravascular footplate with small or severely diseased vessels [37] or embolization of the footplate to the distal vascular bed [38].

Treatment of these occlusions is typically carried by contralateral femoral arterial access with the crossover technique as previously described.

Table 13.4 Common vascular closure devices (VCDs), their mechanism of action, and sheath sizes appropriate for their use.

Device	Mechanism	Sheath size
Perclose	Suture with intravascular component	5–8 Fr Larger sizes possible with preclose technique
Angioseal	Collagen and suture with intravascular component	6 and 8 Fr
Starclose	Extravascular nitinol clip	5 and 6 Fr
Mynx	Extravascular PEG hydrogel plug	5–7 Fr
MANTA	Collagen and suture with intravascular component	14 Fr (10–14 Fr) 18 Fr (15–22 Fr)

Balloon angioplasty is usually sufficient to restore flow. A balloon sized 1 : 1 to the vessel should be used, though a smaller balloon with a better crossing profile may initially be required to traverse the occlusion. A stent is rarely required in cases of CFA injury due to VCDs (see Figure 13.4).

It should be noted that in these cases early referral to a vascular surgical specialist is particularly important. Heroic measures and aggressive escalation of a difficult percutaneous rescue attempt could lead to further complications that can significantly increase patient morbidity. Access site complications are usually easily accessible by surgery and repair can be relatively uncomplicated; therefore, early surgical consultation and a team approach in the treatment of VCD-related complications are essential in treating these patients.

Radial Artery Related Complications

Transradial access (TRA) for PCI has seen a rapid growth in the last 15 years in the United States. National Cardiovascular Data Registry (NCDR) data shows that the number of PCIs performed via the radial artery has increased from 1.2% in 2007 to nearly 50% in 2020. TRA is also being increasingly used in peripheral vascular interventions, with several observational and feasibility studies demonstrating safety and efficacy in carotid, renal, subclavian, common femoral, and iliac artery procedures [39–43]. Its increasing adoption is credited to a lower incidence of access site complications with similar procedural success across the spectrum of coronary disease presentations, collateral blood flow from the ulnar artery which mitigates ischemic complications, and improved patient satisfaction due to early ambulation [44].

(a)　　　　　　　　　　　　　(b)

(c)　　　　　　　　　　　　　(d)

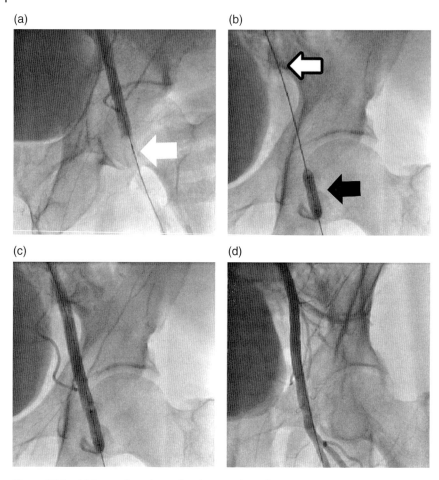

Figure 13.4 (a) Femoral angiography via contralateral access demonstrating acute occlusion of the left CFA (white arrow) after VCD deployment. (b) Through a sheath advanced from the contralateral side (outlined arrow), an angioplasty balloon was advanced across the obstruction over a wire and inflated (black arrow). (c) Angiography with the balloon inflated confirms 1 : 1 sizing. (d) Final angiography demonstrates resolution of obstruction and brisk distal flow.

Radial Artery Spasm

Radial artery spasm (RAS) occurs in about 10% of TRA procedures [45], and contributes to patient discomfort or even procedural failure leading to access site crossover. Prevention of spasm is of utmost importance: measures include administration of spasmolytic "cocktails" and adequate sedation and analgesia, as well as the use of hydrophilic sheaths [46, 47]. Some advocate the use of long sheaths to "bypass" the radial artery during equipment exchanges; however, evidence to support their use has not been conclusive [48, 49].

When it does occur, radial spasm can be treated with intraarterial vasodilators like nitroglycerin or verapamil, deeper patient sedation, and appropriate analgesia. Exchanging for smaller sheaths and catheters may also be effective. In addition, patience of the part of the operator is important as radial spasm often improves after allowing for time without equipment manipulation. In especially severe cases, axillary nerve block, deep sedation, or even general anesthesia may be required for sheath removal [50, 51]. Care should be taken to avoid applying excessive force in removing radial arterial sheaths in the presence of RAS, as this may result in radial artery transection or avulsion.

Radial Artery Occlusion

Radial artery occlusion (RAO) is the most common complication of TRA, but is rarely associated with adverse clinical consequences given the dual blood supply of the hand, and is often underdiagnosed as it is usually asymptomatic. Risk factors for RAO include older age, female gender, smaller body size, and sheath-artery mismatch [52]. In a 66-study meta-analysis, the incidence of RAO was found to be 11% with 6 Fr sheaths and 2% with 5 Fr sheaths, and on average decreased from 7.7% in the first 24 hours after the index procedure to 5.5% at 1 week due to spontaneous recanalization. Rates of RAO were lower with PCI (4.5%) compared to diagnostic angiography (8.8%), likely due to routine use of antithrombotic therapy with PCI.

Prevention of RAO is focused on periprocedural anticoagulation and postprocedural "patent hemostasis." Unfractionated heparin during transradial catheterization has been proven to reduce rates of RAO in a dose-dependent fashion [53], though bivalirudin or low molecular weight heparin (LMWH) has also been shown to be effective [54]. "Patent hemostasis" after sheath removal has also been shown to decrease rates of RAO compared to traditional compression, by preserving antegrade arterial flow while maintaining hemostasis [55]. Antegrade flow through the radial artery should be confirmed by observing a waveform on plethysmography while manually occluding the ulnar artery.

If RAO is suspected, confirmation should be sought with plethysmography or duplex arterial ultrasonography. The treatment strategy is based on presence of symptoms and acuity of the diagnosis. In the absence of symptoms, radial artery recanalization is not favored since clinical consequences of RAO in the presence of a patent ulnar artery are minimal. In the acute setting, transient ulnar compression has been described as a noninvasive method to recanalize the radial artery [56]. One single center observational study found anticoagulation with LMWH for four weeks in patients with symptomatic RAO resulted in recanalization of the artery in 87% of cases [57].

Bleeding Complications

Access site related bleeding usually results in hematoma formation in the forearm or upper arm. Hematomas may be categorized using the EASY (Early Discharge After Transradial Stenting of Coronary Arteries) grading system (Figure 13.5): grade I, ≤5cm (local hematoma, superficial); grade II, ≤10cm (hematoma with moderate muscular infiltration); grade III, >10cm below the elbow – forearm hematoma and muscular infiltration; grade IV, above the elbow; and grade V, anywhere with ischemic threat (compartment syndrome). Hematoma grades I and II are usually related to puncture site bleeding, while grades III and IV usually result from inadvertent wire perforation or catheter damage of the artery upstream from the access site. Timely recognition of transradial-related hematomas is of utmost importance to prevent progression to compartment syndrome, a rare (0.004%) but limb-threatening complication [58]. Small hematomas near the access site should prompt evaluation of the hemostatic compression device position, and usually placement of a pressure dressing or another compression device may be needed. For larger, grade III or IV hematomas, a sphygmomanometer should be

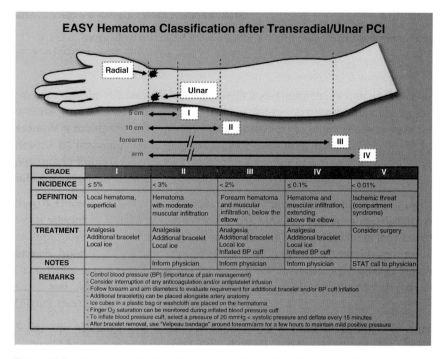

EASY Hematoma Classification after Transradial/Ulnar PCI

GRADE	I	II	III	IV	V
INCIDENCE	≤ 5%	< 3%	< 2%	≤ 0.1%	< 0.01%
DEFINITION	Local hematoma, superficial	Hematoma with moderate muscular infiltration	Forearm hematoma and muscular infiltration, below the elbow	Hematoma and muscular infiltration, extending above the elbow	Ischemic threat (compartment syndrome)
TREATMENT	Analgesia Additional bracelet Local ice	Analgesia Additional bracelet Local ice	Analgesia Additional bracelet Local ice Inflated BP cuff	Analgesia Additional bracelet Local ice Inflated BP cuff	Consider surgery
NOTES		Inform physician	Inform physician	Inform physician	STAT call to physician
REMARKS	- Control blood pressure (BP) (importance of pain management) - Consider interruption of any anticoagulation and/or antiplatelet infusion - Follow forearm and arm diameters to evaluate requirement for additional bracelet and/or BP cuff inflation - Additional bracelet(s) can be placed alongside artery anatomy - Ice cubes in a plastic bag or washcloth are placed on the hematoma - Finger O$_2$ saturation can be monitored during inflated blood pressure cuff - To inflate blood pressure cuff, select a pressure of 20 mmHg < systolic pressure and deflate every 15 minutes - After bracelet removal, use "Velpeau bandage" around forearm/arm for a few hours to maintain mild positive pressure			

Figure 13.5 Hematoma classification proposed in the Early Discharge After Transradial Stenting of Coronary Arteries (EASY) trial.

immediately inflated proximal to the hematoma to a pressure 20 mmHg below systolic blood pressure to achieve hemostasis while compression dressings are being placed, then deflated gradually over 30–60 minutes. Worsening symptoms of hand pain, paresthesia, and pallor in the presence of a tense forearm compartment should prompt urgent surgical consultation.

References

1 Muller, D.W., Shamir, K.J., Ellis, S.G., and Topol, E.J. (1992). Peripheral vascular complications after conventional and complex percutaneous coronary interventional procedures. *Am. J. Cardiol.* 69: 63–68.

2 Metz, D., Meyer, P., Touati, C. et al. (1997). Comparison of 6F with 7F and 8F guiding catheters for elective coronary angioplasty: results of a prospective, multicenter, randomized trial. *Am. Heart J.* 134: 131–137.

3 Arora, N., Matheny, M.E., Sepke, C., and Resnic, F.S. (2007). A propensity analysis of the risk of vascular complications after cardiac catheterization procedures with the use of vascular closure devices. *Am. Heart J.* 153: 606–611.

4 Chase, A.J., Fretz, E.B., Warburton, W.P. et al. (2008). Association of the arterial access site at angioplasty with transfusion and mortality: the MORTAL study (mortality benefit of reduced transfusion after percutaneous coronary intervention via the arm or leg). *Heart* 94: 1019–1025.

5 Kinnaird, T.D., Stabile, E., Mintz, G.S. et al. (2003). Incidence, predictors, and prognostic implications of bleeding and blood transfusion following percutaneous coronary interventions. *Am. J. Cardiol.* 92: 930–935.

6 Feit, F., Voeltz, M.D., Attubato, M.J. et al. (2007). Predictors and impact of major hemorrhage on mortality following percutaneous coronary intervention from the REPLACE-2 trial. *Am. J. Cardiol.* 100: 1364–1369.

7 Yatskar, L., Selzer, F., Feit, F. et al. (2007). Access site hematoma requiring blood transfusion predicts mortality in patients undergoing percutaneous coronary intervention: data from the National Heart, Lung, and Blood Institute Dynamic Registry. *Catheter. Cardiovasc. Interv.* 69: 961–966.

8 Piper, W.D., Malenka, D.J., Ryan, T.J. et al. (2003). Predicting vascular complications in percutaneous coronary interventions. *Am. Heart J.* 145: 1022–1029.

9 Aguirre, F.V., Topol, E.J., Ferguson, J.J. et al. (1995). Bleeding complications with the chimeric antibody to platelet glycoprotein IIb/IIIa integrin in patients undergoing percutaneous coronary intervention. *Circulation* 91: 2882–2890.

10 Friedman, H.Z., Cragg, D.R., Glazier, S.M. et al. (1994). Randomized prospective evaluation of prolonged versus abbreviated intravenous heparin therapy after coronary angioplasty. *J. Am. Coll. Cardiol.* 24: 1214–1219.

11 Mandak, J.S., Blankenship, J.C., Gardner, L.H. et al. (1998). Modifiable risk factors for vascular access site complications in the IMPACT II trial of angioplasty with versus without eptifibatide. *J. Am. Coll. Cardiol.* 31: 1518–1524.

12 Lincoff, A.M., Tcheng, J.E., Califf, R.M. et al. (1997). Standard versus low-dose weight-adjusted heparin in patients treated with the platelet glycoprotein IIb/IIIa receptor antibody fragment abciximab (c7E3 Fab) during percutaneous coronary revascularization. *Am. J. Cardiol.* 79: 286–291.

13 Kent, K.C., Moscucci, M., Mansour, K.A. et al. (1994). Retroperitoneal hematoma after cardiac catheterization: prevalence, risk factors, and optimal management. *J. Vasc. Surg.* 20: 905–913.

14 Trimarchi, S., Smith, D.E., Share, D. et al. (2010). Retroperitoneal hematoma after percutaneous coronary intervention: prevalence, risk factors, management, outcomes, and predictors of mortality: a report from the BMC2 (Blue Cross Blue Shield of Michigan Cardiovascular Consortium) registry. *J. Am. Coll. Cardiol. Intv.* 3: 845–850.

15 Farouque, H.O., Tremmel, J.A., Shabari, F.R. et al. (2005). Risk factors for the development of retroperitoneal hematoma after percutaneous coronary intervention in the era of glycoprotein IIb/IIIa inhibitors and vascular closure devices. *J. Am. Coll. Cardiol.* 45: 363–368.

16 Duerig, T.W. and Wholey, M. (2002). A comparison of balloon- and self-expanding stents. *Minim. Invasive Ther. Allied Technol.* 11: 173–178.

17 Katzenschlager, R., Ugurluoglu, A., Ahmadi, A. et al. (1995). Incidence of pseudoaneurysm after diagnostic and therapeutic angiography. *Radiology* 195: 463–466.

18 Lumsden, A.B., Miller, J.M., Kosinski, A.S. et al. (1994). A prospective evaluation of surgically treated groin complications following percutaneous cardiac procedures. *Am. Surg.* 60: 132–137.

19 Kim, D., Orron, D.E., Skillman, J.J. et al. (1992). Role of superficial femoral artery puncture in the development of pseudoaneurysm and arteriovenous fistula complicating percutaneous transfemoral cardiac catheterization. *Cathet. Cardiovasc. Diagn.* 25: 91–97.

20 Waksman, R., King, S.B., Douglas, J.S. et al. (1995). Predictors of groin complications after balloon and new-device coronary intervention. *Am. J. Cardiol.* 75: 886–889.

21 Fellmeth, B.D., Roberts, A.C., Bookstein, J.J. et al. (1991). Postangiographic femoral artery injuries: nonsurgical repair with US-guided compression. *Radiology* 178: 671–675.

22 Feld, R., Patton, G.M., Carabasi, R.A. et al. (1992). Treatment of iatrogenic femoral artery injuries with ultrasound-guided compression. *J. Vasc. Surg.* 16: 832–840.

23 Hajarizadeh, H., LaRosa, C.R., Cardullo, P. et al. (1995). Ultrasound-guided compression of iatrogenic femoral pseudoaneurysm failure, recurrence, and long-term results. *J. Vasc. Surg.* 22: 425–433.

24 Dean, S.M., Olin, J.W., Piedmonte, M. et al. (1996). Ultrasound-guided compression closure of postcatheterization pseudoaneurysms during concurrent anticoagulation: a review of seventy-seven patients. *J. Vasc. Surg.* 23: 28–35.

25 Chatterjee, T., Do, D.D., Kaufmann, U. et al. (1996). Ultrasound-guided compression repair for treatment of femoral artery pseudoaneurysm: acute and follow-up results. *Cathet. Cardiovasc. Diagn.* 38: 335–340.

26 Eisenberg, L., Paulson, E.K., Kliewer, M.A. et al. (1999). Sonographically guided compression repair of pseudoaneurysms: further experience from a single institution. *Am. J. Roentgenol.* 173: 1567–1573.

27 Paulson, E.K., Nelson, R.C., Mayes, C.E. et al. (2001). Sonographically guided thrombin injection of latrogenic femoral pseudoaneurysms. *Am. J. Roentgenol.* 177: 309–316.

28 La Perna, L., Olin, J.W., Goines, D. et al. (2000). Ultrasound-guided thrombin injection for the treatment of postcatheterization pseudoaneurysms. *Circulation* 102: 2391–2395.

29 Khoury, M., Rebecca, A., Greene, K. et al. (2002). Duplex scanning–guided thrombin injection for the treatment of iatrogenic pseudoaneurysms. *J. Vasc. Surg.* 35: 517–521.

30 Friedman, S.G. (2002). Ultrasound-guided thrombin injection is the treatment of choice for femoral pseudoaneurysms. *Arch. Surg.* 137: 462.

31 Waigand, J., Uhlich, F., Gross, C.M. et al. (1999). Percutaneous treatment of pseudoaneurysms and arteriovenous fistulas after invasive vascular procedures. *Catheter. Cardiovasc. Interv.* 47: 157–164.

32 Thalhammer, C., Kirchherr, A.S., Uhlich, F. et al. (2000). Postcatheterization pseudoaneurysms and arteriovenous fistulas: repair with percutaneous implantation of endovascular covered stents 1. *Radiology* 214: 127–131.

33 Morgan, R. and Belli, A.M. (2003). Current treatment methods for postcatheterization pseudoaneurysms. *J. Vasc. Interv. Radiol.* 14: 697–710.

34 Kelm, M., Perings, S.M., Jax, T. et al. (2002). Incidence and clinical outcome of iatrogenic femoral arteriovenous fistulas: implications for risk stratification and treatment. *J. Am. Coll. Cardiol.* 40: 291–297.

35 Perings, S.M., Kelm, M., Jax, T., and Strauer, B.E. (2003). A prospective study on incidence and risk factors of arteriovenous fistulae following transfemoral cardiac catheterization. *Int. J. Cardiol.* 88: 223–228.

36 Archie, M. and Farley, S. (2018). Possible mechanism for common femoral artery occlusion with the Perclose suture device. *Ann. Vasc. Surg.* 49: 309.e17–309.e21.

37 Srinivasan, M., Kariyanna, P.T., Smith, J. et al. (2020). Angio-seal vascular closure related acute limb ischemia: a case report. *Am. J. Med. Case Rep.* 8: 49–52.

38 Lasam, G., Oaks, J.B., and Brensilver, J. (2017). Angio-Seal™ embolization: a rare etiology of an acute distal limb ischemia. *Case Rep. Vasc. Med.* 2017: 1–3.

39 Patel, T., Shah, S., Ranjan, A. et al. (2010). Contralateral transradial approach for carotid artery stenting: a feasibility study. *Catheter. Cardiovasc. Interv.* 75: 268–275.

40 Folmar, J., Sachar, R., and Mann, T. (2007). Transradial approach for carotid artery stenting: a feasibility study. *Catheter. Cardiovasc. Interv.* 69: 355–361.

41 Trani, C., Burzotta, F., Tommasino, A., and Giammarinaro, M. (2009). Transradial approach to treat superficial femoral artery in-stent restenosis. *Catheter. Cardiovasc. Interv.* 74: 494–498.

42 Sanghvi, K., Kurian, D., and Coppola, J. (2008). Transradial intervention of iliac and superficial femoral artery disease is feasible. *J. Interv. Cardiol.* 21: 385–387.

43 Trani, C., Tommasino, A., and Burzotta, F. (2009). Transradial renal stenting: why and how. *Catheter. Cardiovasc. Interv.* 74: 951–956.

44 Ferrante, G., Rao, S.V., Jüni, P. et al. (2016). Radial versus femoral access for coronary interventions across the entire spectrum of patients with coronary artery disease: a meta-analysis of randomized trials. *J. Am. Coll. Cardiol. Intv.* 9: 1419–1434.

45 Goldberg, S.L., Renslo, R., Sinow, R., and French, W.J. (1998). Learning curve in the use of the radial artery as vascular access in the performance of percutaneous transluminal coronary angioplasty. *Cathet. Cardiovasc. Diagn.* 44: 147–152.

46 Caputo, R.P., Tremmel, J.A., Rao, S. et al. (2011). Transradial arterial access for coronary and peripheral procedures: executive summary by the Transradial Committee of the SCAI. *Catheter. Cardiovasc. Interv.* 78: 823–839.

47 Kiemeneij, F., Fraser, D., Slagboom, T. et al. (2003). Hydrophilic coating aids radial sheath withdrawal and reduces patient discomfort following transradial coronary intervention: a randomized double-blind comparison of coated and uncoated sheaths. *Catheter. Cardiovasc. Interv.* 59: 161–164.

48 Caussin, C., Gharbi, M., Durier, C. et al. (2010). Reduction in spasm with a long hydrophylic transradial sheath. *Catheter. Cardiovasc. Interv.* 76: 668–672.

49 Dieter, R.S., Akef, A., and Wolff, M. (2003). Eversion endarterectomy complicating radial artery access for left heart catheterization. *Catheter. Cardiovasc. Interv.* 58: 478–480.

50 Eltahawy, E.A. and Cooper, C.J. (2010). Managing radial access vascular complications. *Cardiac Inte Today* 4: 46–49.

51 Pullakhandam, N.S., Yang, Z.-j., Thomas, S., and Wasenko, J. (2006). Unusual complication of transradial catheterization. *Anesth. Analg.* 103: 794–795.

52 Rathore, S., Stables, R.H., Pauriah, M. et al. (2010). A randomized comparison of TR band and radistop hemostatic compression devices after transradial coronary intervention. *Catheter. Cardiovasc. Interv.* 76: 660–667.

53 Pancholy, S.B. (2009). Comparison of the effect of intra-arterial versus intravenous heparin on radial artery occlusion after transradial catheterization. *Am. J. Cardiol.* 104: 1083–1085.

54 Plante, S., Cantor, W.J., Goldman, L. et al. (2010). Comparison of bivalirudin versus heparin on radial artery occlusion after transradial catheterization. *Catheter. Cardiovasc. Interv.* 76: 654–658.

55 Pancholy, S., Coppola, J., Patel, T., and Roke-Thomas, M. (2008). Prevention of radial artery occlusion—patent hemostasis evaluation trial (PROPHET study): a randomized comparison of traditional versus patency documented hemostasis after transradial catheterization. *Catheter. Cardiovasc. Interv.* 72: 335–340.

56 Bernat, I., Bertrand, O.F., Rokyta, R. et al. (2011). Efficacy and safety of transient ulnar artery compression to recanalize acute radial artery occlusion after transradial catheterization. *Am. J. Cardiol.* 107: 1698–1701.

57 Zankl, A.R., Andrassy, M., Volz, C. et al. (2010). Radial artery thrombosis following transradial coronary angiography: incidence and rationale for treatment of symptomatic patients with low-molecular-weight heparins. *Clin. Res. Cardiol.* 99: 841–847.

58 Tizón-Marcos, H. and Barbeau, G.R. (2008). Incidence of compartment syndrome of the arm in a large series of transradial approach for coronary procedures. *J. Interv. Cardiol.* 21: 380–384.

14

Acute Deep Vein Thrombosis

Vishal Kapur and Sagar Goyal

Division of Cardiology, The Zena and Michael A. Weiner Cardiovascular Institute, Icahn School of Medicine at Mount Sinai, New York, NY, USA

Introduction

Acute deep venous thrombosis (DVT) is a life-threatening condition that can have serious potential consequences. Early diagnosis and treatment form the cornerstone of disease management. The introduction of direct oral anticoagulation and advancement in invasive techniques have improved the outcomes in this subgroup of patients. This chapter overviews the comprehensive management of patients with acute DVT.

Accurate diagnosis of lower-extremity DVT is extremely important, given the potentially fatal risks of untreated DVT in the form of pulmonary embolism (PE) and the risks of anticoagulation used for its treatment (e.g. major or life-threatening bleeding).

Lower-extremity DVT and PE are two manifestations of venous thromboembolism (VTE). The diagnosis of VTE is made in a sequence of steps including assessment of the pretest probability, followed by D-dimer testing and imaging as appropriate (Figure 14.1).

Overall, VTE can be excluded in 29% (95% CI, 20–40%) of patients with suspected DVT and 28% (95% CI, 20–37%) of those with suspected PE using diagnostic algorithms including pretest probability assessment and D-dimer testing (Figure 14.1) [2, 3]. The remaining patients require compression ultrasonography or computed tomography pulmonary angiography (CTPA) to determine whether VTE is present [4–6].

When VTE is diagnosed, immediate initiation of anticoagulant therapy is imperative.

Endovascular Interventions: A Step-by-Step Approach, First Edition. Edited by Jose M. Wiley, Cristina Sanina, George D. Dangas, and Prakash Krishnan.

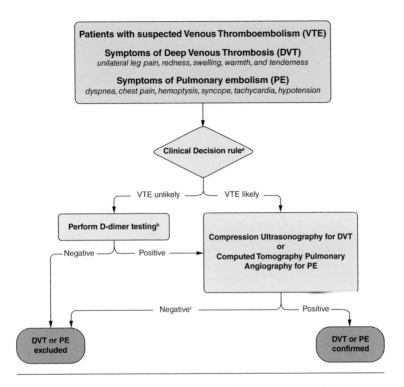

[a]Wells score for suspected DVT and Wells score or revised Geneva score for suspected PE.

[b]Age-adjusted D-dimer threshold, calculated as the patient's age multiplied by 10 ng/ml (fibrinogen-equivalent units) for patients older than 50 years with suspected PE.

[c]Repeat compression ultrasonography 1 week after initially normal findings in patients with high clinical probability and positive D-dimer levels if initial imaging was not whole-leg ultrasonography.

Figure 14.1 Diagnostic management of patients with suspected DVT or PE [1].

Treatment Strategy

There are three phases of VTE treatment: the initial (first 5–10 days), long-term (from the end of acute treatment to 3–6 months), and extended (beyond 3–6 months) periods. The benefits of anticoagulation, including prevention of clot extension, PE, recurrent VTE, hemodynamic collapse, and death, should be carefully weighed against the risk of bleeding to determine the choice of anticoagulant and the duration of therapy (Figure 14.2).

VTE events are often classified as being "provoked" by a transient or persistent risk factor or as "unprovoked" in the absence of any identifiable risk factors for VTE to estimate the risk of recurrent VTE and guide decisions on treatment

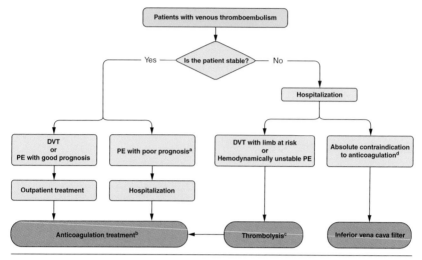

Figure 14.2   Approach to initial treatment of venous thromboembolism (onset through days 5–10).

duration [7]. In patients with VTE provoked by surgery, the risk of recurrence after treatment is low (<1% after one year and 3% after five years); those with VTE caused by a nonsurgical transient risk factor, such as immobilization, pregnancy, or estrogen therapy, have an intermediate risk of recurrent VTE (5% after one year and 15% after five years) [8]. In both situations, anticoagulation is recommended for only three months, as previous randomized trials showed that major bleeding risk during extended anticoagulant treatment beyond this period outweighed the risk of recurrent VTE [5, 6, 8, 9]. Patients with cancer-associated VTE have a high risk of recurrence (15% annualized), and therapy may be given until the cancer is cured [5, 6, 8].

When a patient does not have any identifiable risk factors for VTE, the event is classified as unprovoked.

Patients with a first unprovoked VTE have a high risk of recurrence of VTE (10% after one year and 30% at five years) and should therefore receive indefinite therapy unless the bleeding risk is high [5, 6, 8]. The risk in men is at least double than that in women (Figure 14.3).

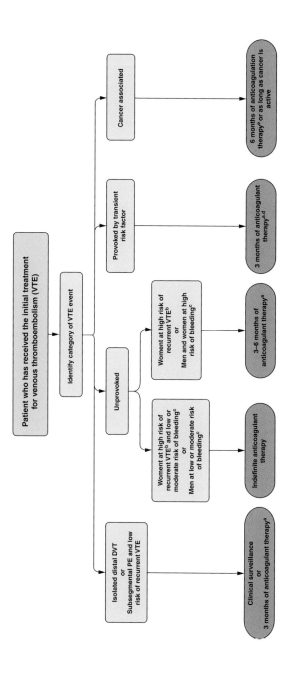

Abbreviations: DVT, Deep Venous Thrombosis; PE, Pulmonary Embolism

[a] Anticoagulation with direct oral anticoagulants (rivaroxaban or apixaban, or initial low-molecular-weight heparin followed by dabigatran or edoxaban). Vitamin K antagonists are indicated for patients with a creatinine clearance of less than 30 mL/min and those with concomitant use of potent P-glycoprotein inhibitors or cytochrome P450 3A4 inhibitors or inducers.

[b] If transient risk factor is nonsurgical (eg, immobilization, pregnancy, or estrogen therapy), extended treatment can be considered given the safety profile of direct oral anticoagulants.

[c] Edoxaban or low-molecular-weight heparin.

[d] Low-risk women according to the HERDOO2 rule.

[e] Bleeding risk according to HAS-BLED score. HAS-BLED categorizes patients into low (score, 0–2) or high (score, 23) risk.

Figure 14.3 Approach to long-term and extended treatment of VTE (after initial treatment).

Initial and Long-Term Treatment of VTE

Oral Anticoagulants

Over the past decade, direct oral anticoagulants (DOACs), including the direct thrombin inhibitor dabigatran and the factor Xa inhibitors rivaroxaban, apixaban, and edoxaban, have been studied and are now recommended by the 2016 American College of Chest Physicians and the 2014 and 2017 European Society of Cardiology guidelines for both DVT and PE [5, 8, 9]. However, vitamin K antagonists remain the preferred treatment for patients with severe renal impairment. Similarly, DOACs are generally avoided in patients with concomitant use of potent P-glycoprotein inhibitors or cytochrome P4503A4 inhibitors or inducers, including azole antimycotics (e.g. ketoconazole), several protease inhibitors used for human immunodeficiency virus treatment (e.g. ritonavir), and antiepileptic drugs (in particular, phenytoin and carbamazepine), because they can alter plasma levels of DOACs.

Compared with initial LMWH followed by long-term VKA treatment, DOACs are noninferior for recurrent VTE and are associated with a lower risk of major bleeding, as defined by the International Society on Thrombosis and Hemostasis [10] (absolute risk, 1.1% vs. 1.8%; risk ratio, 0.62; 95% CI, 0.45–0.85) in the first months of VTE treatment [11]. All-cause mortality and case-fatality rates of recurrent VTE or major bleeding with DOACs are comparable with rates with LMWH/VKA [12]. DOAC therapy is currently more expensive than treatment with VKAs. Monthly costs range between $333 and $419 with DOACs, whereas generic VKAs cost $8 per month [13].

These agents were developed according to two different regimens for the treatment of VTE (Table 14.1) [14–19]. The single-drug approach consists of an initial treatment period with high-dose DOACs followed by a maintenance dose of the same agent with no need for parenteral anticoagulation. The sequential approach includes an initial treatment with LWMH or fondaparinux for 5–10 days followed by a maintenance dose of DOACs. Apixaban and rivaroxaban have been developed according to the single-drug approach, and dabigatran and edoxaban have been developed according to the sequential approach [20].

Thrombolysis

Catheter-directed thrombolysis as initial treatment of acute DVT is currently recommended only for patients with threatened limb loss [8]. A Cochrane review including patients with acute proximal DVT showed that thrombolysis plus anticoagulation compared with anticoagulation alone may reduce postthrombotic syndrome by one-third (risk ratio, 0.66; 95% CI, 0.53–0.81) [21]. However,

Table 14.1 Parenteral and oral anticoagulants.

Name	Dosage
Parenteral agents	
Unfractionated heparin	Sodium heparin: 80 IU/kg followed by 18 IU/kg per hour continuous infusion
Enoxaparin sc	1 mg/kg every 12 h or 1.5 mg.kg once per day
Fondaparinux sc	5 mg (wt <50 kg); 7.5 mg (wt 50–75 kg); 10 mg (wt >100 kg) once per day
Dalteparin sc	100 IU/kg every 12 h or 200 IU/kg once per day
Tinzaparin sc	175 IU/kg per day
Nadroparin sc	86 IU/kg every 12 h or 171 IU/kg once per day
Oral agents	
Rivaroxaban	15 mg twice daily for 21 d then 20 mg once daily
Apixaban	10 mg twice a day for 1 wk then 5 mg twice daily
Dabigatran	150 mg po twice day after 5–7 d of parenteral treatment
Edoxaban	60 mg once a day for 5–7 d after parenteral treatment
Vitamin K antagonist	INR adjusted dosage

thrombolysis appeared to have no effect on the occurrence of PE, recurrent DVT, or death and, moreover, has an increased bleeding risk [11]. Results did not differ between thrombolytic agents and route of administration (systemic vs. locoregional vs. catheter-directed) [21]. The recent randomized trial ATTRACT confirmed these findings, as pharmacomechanical catheter-directed thrombolysis (i.e. local administration of thrombolytic agent with concomitant thrombus aspiration or maceration) compared with anticoagulation alone did not lead to better results with regard to VTE recurrence or mortality and led to an increased risk of major bleeding in the first 10 days [22]. Notably, the occurrence of postthrombotic syndrome after 24 months was similar in both treatment groups, suggesting no role for catheter-directed thrombolysis in the routine management of DVT [22].

Vena Cava Filters

Inferior vena cava filters may be used in patients with proximal DVT or PE who have an absolute contraindication to anticoagulant therapy but are not recommended in those who can receive anticoagulation [5, 6, 8, 9]. The use of a retrievable inferior vena cava filter for three months in addition to standard anticoagulation compared with anticoagulation alone was recently evaluated in a randomized trial including 399 hospitalized patients with severe acute PE [23]. There was no reduction in recurrent PE or death at three- and six-month follow-up [23].

Compression Stockings

The use of graduated compression stockings after acute proximal DVT does not reduce the incidence of postthrombotic syndrome compared with placebo or no stockings [24]. Accordingly, compression stockings are recommended only as symptomatic treatment in patients with acute or chronic symptoms, such as swelling and discomfort [5, 6, 8, 9].

Cancer-Associated VTE

Cancer patients have an increased risk of both recurrent VTE and bleeding complications. The 2016 American College of Chest Physicians and the 2014 and 2017 European Society of Cardiology guidelines recommend long-term daily subcutaneous LMWH as the first-choice drug in patients with cancer-associated VTE [6, 8, 9].

The 2018 guidance of the International Society on Thrombosis and Hemostasis suggests specific DOACs (edoxaban or rivaroxaban) for treatment of cancer-associated VTE in patients with a low risk of bleeding and no drug–drug interactions with DOACs [25].

In the United States, edoxaban costs $337, rivaroxaban $333, and dalteparin $3527 per month [13], so in addition to having similar efficacy, DOACs are less expensive than dalteparin.

Isolated Distal DVT

The 2016 American College of Chest Physicians guidelines suggest that ultrasound surveillance of isolated distal DVT to monitor for thrombus extension to the proximal veins is preferred over anticoagulation in patients with a low risk of extension [8].

Extended Treatment

Unprovoked VTE

Extended treatment for long-term prevention of recurrent VTE is indicated for patients with unprovoked VTE, unless bleeding risk is high.

Negative (normal) D-dimer levels measured serially after stopping anticoagulation are associated with a low risk of recurrent VTE and may be used to guide the decision to stop anticoagulant treatment in women but not in men, because they have an unacceptably high risk of recurrent VTE even if D-dimer levels are normal (9.7% per patient-year; 95% CI, 6.7–13.7%) [26, 27]. However, the requirement for measurement of D-dimers while not receiving treatment, the use of different cut-offs to define a normal test result, and the use of different D-dimer assays in the validation studies call into question the utility of this approach.

Oral Anticoagulants

The 2016 American College of Chest Physicians and the 2014 and 2017 European Society of Cardiology guidelines suggest extended therapy with DOACs over VKAs or low-dose aspirin in patients without cancer [6, 8, 9]. Compared with placebo or aspirin, extended therapy with DOACs or VKAs significantly reduces the risk of recurrent VTE [14, 28–30]. Compared with VKAs, dabigatran and edoxaban are as effective and are associated with a lower risk of major bleeding (0.9% vs. 1.8%; HR, 0.52; 95% CI, 0.27–1.02 for dabigatran; 0.3% vs. 0.7%; HR, 0.45; 95% CI, 0.22–0.92 for edoxaban) [14, 30, 31]. In contrast to extended treatment with VKAs, the introduction of DOACs has enabled extended anticoagulant therapy at a lower dosage, as apixaban and rivaroxaban at prophylactic dosages (10 mg once daily and 2.5 mg twice daily, respectively) are associated with similar efficacy as at therapeutic dosages (20 mg once daily and 5 mg twice daily, respectively) and a bleeding risk comparable with placebo and aspirin (absolute risk of major bleeding <0.5% per year) [29, 32].

Conclusion

When left untreated, VTE was associated with early recurrences (29%) and death (26%) in landmark studies [33, 34]. Based on this evidence, early anticoagulant treatment should be started in patients with suspected VTE who are estimated to not be at high risk for bleeding while they wait for diagnostic confirmation [8, 35].

Pivotal studies showed that failure to rapidly receive therapeutic anticoagulation [36, 37] and time spent while receiving subtherapeutic anticoagulation are both associated with recurrent VTEs [38]. Thus, the availability of anticoagulants with rapid onset of action and predictable dose-effect response are essential for reducing early adverse effects.

References

1 Tritschler, T., Kraaijpoel, N., Le Gal, G., and Wells, P.S. (2018). Venous thromboembolism: advances in diagnosis and treatment. *JAMA* 320 (15): 1583.

2 Geersing, G.J., Zuithoff, N.P.A., Kearon, C. et al. (2014). Exclusion of deep vein thrombosis using the Wells rule in clinically important subgroups: individual patient data meta-analysis. *BMJ* 348 (3): g1340.

3 van Es, N., van der Hulle, T., van Es, J. et al. (2016). Wells rule and d -dimer testing to rule out pulmonary embolism: a systematic review and individual-patient data meta-analysis. *Ann. Intern. Med.* 165 (4): 253.

4 Bates, S.M., Jaeschke, R., Stevens, S.M. et al. (2012). Diagnosis of DVT. *Chest* 141 (2): e351S–e418S.

5 Mazzolai, L., Aboyans, V., Ageno, W. et al. (2018). Diagnosis and management of acute deep vein thrombosis: a joint consensus document from the European Society of Cardiology working groups of aorta and peripheral vascular diseases and pulmonary circulation and right ventricular function. *Eur. Heart J.* 39 (47): 4208–4218.

6 Authors/Task Force Members, Konstantinides, S.V., Torbicki, A. et al. (2014). 2014 ESC Guidelines on the diagnosis and management of acute pulmonary embolism. *Eur. Heart J.* 35 (43): 3033–3080.

7 Kearon, C., Ageno, W., Cannegieter, S.C. et al. (2016). Categorization of patients as having provoked or unprovoked venous thromboembolism: guidance from the SSC of ISTH. *J. Thromb. Haemost.* 14 (7): 1480–1483.

8 Kearon, C., Akl, E.A., Ornelas, J. et al. (2016). Antithrombotic therapy for VTE disease. *Chest* 149 (2): 315–352.

9 Schulman, S., Konstantinides, S., Hu, Y. et al. (2020). Venous thromboembolic diseases: diagnosis, management and thrombophilia testing: observations on NICE Guideline [NG158]. *Thromb. Haemost.* 120 (8): 1143–1146.

10 Schulman, S., Kearon, C., and The subcommittee on control of anticoagulation of the scientific and standardization committee of the international society on thrombosis and haemostasis (2005). Definition of major bleeding in clinical investigations of antihemostatic medicinal products in non-surgical patients: definitions of major bleeding in clinical studies. *J. Thromb. Haemost.* 3 (4): 692–694.

11 Gómez-Outes, A., Terleira-Fernández, A.I., Lecumberri, R. et al. (2014). Direct oral anticoagulants in the treatment of acute venous thromboembolism: a systematic review and meta-analysis. *Thromb. Res.* 134 (4): 774–782.

12 Gómez-Outes, A., Lecumberri, R., Suárez-Gea, M.L. et al. (2015). Case fatality rates of recurrent thromboembolism and bleeding in patients receiving direct oral anticoagulants for the initial and extended treatment of venous thromboembolism: a systematic review. *J. Cardiovasc. Pharmacol. Ther.* 20 (5): 490–500.

13 (2018). Drugs for treatment and prevention of venous thromboembolism. *Med. Lett. Drugs Ther.* 60 (1542): 41–48.

14 The Hokusai-VTE Investigators (2013). Edoxaban versus warfarin for the treatment of symptomatic venous thromboembolism. *N. Engl. J. Med.* 369 (15): 1406–1415.

15 Agnelli, G., Buller, H.R., Cohen, A. et al. (2013). Oral Apixaban for the treatment of acute venous thromboembolism. *N. Engl. J. Med.* 369 (9): 799–808.

16 Bauersachs, R., Berkowitz, S.D., Brenner, B. et al. (2010). Oral rivaroxaban for symptomatic venous thromboembolism. *N. Engl. J. Med.* 363 (26): 2499–2510.

17 Büller, H.R., Prins, M.H., Lensing, A.W.A. et al. (2012). Oral rivaroxaban for the treatment of symptomatic pulmonary embolism. *N. Engl. J. Med.* 366 (14): 1287–1297.

18 Schulman, S., Kearon, C., Kakkar, A.K. et al. (2009). Dabigatran versus warfarin in the treatment of acute venous thromboembolism. *N. Engl. J. Med.* 361 (24): 2342–2352.

19 Schulman, S., Kakkar, A.K., Goldhaber, S.Z. et al. (2014). Treatment of acute venous thromboembolism with dabigatran or warfarin and pooled analysis. *Circulation* 129 (7): 764–772.

20 Becattini, C. and Agnelli, G. (2016). Treatment of venous thromboembolism with new anticoagulant agents. *J. Am. Coll. Cardiol.* 67 (16): 1941–1955.

21 Watson, L., Broderick, C., and Armon, M.P. (2016). Thrombolysis for acute deep vein thrombosis. (ed. Cochrane Vascular Group). *Cochrane Database of Systematic Reviews.* http://doi.wiley.com/10.1002/14651858.CD002783.pub4.

22 Vedantham, S., Goldhaber, S.Z., Julian, J.A. et al. (2017). Pharmacomechanical catheter-directed thrombolysis for deep-vein thrombosis. *N. Engl. J. Med.* 377 (23): 2240–2252.

23 Mismetti, P., Laporte, S., Pellerin, O. et al. (2015). Effect of a retrievable inferior vena cava filter plus anticoagulation vs anticoagulation alone on risk of recurrent pulmonary embolism: a randomized clinical trial. *JAMA* 313 (16): 1627.

24 Subbiah, R., Aggarwal, V., Zhao, H. et al. (2016). Effect of compression stockings on post thrombotic syndrome in patients with deep vein thrombosis: a meta-analysis of randomised controlled trials. *Lancet Haematol.* 3 (6): e293–e300.

25 Khorana, A.A., Noble, S., Lee, A.Y.Y. et al. (2018). Role of direct oral anticoagulants in the treatment of cancer-associated venous thromboembolism: guidance from the SSC of the ISTH. *J. Thromb. Haemost.* 16 (9): 1891–1894.

26 Kearon, C., Spencer, F.A., O'Keeffe, D. et al. (2015). d -Dimer testing to select patients with a first unprovoked venous thromboembolism who can stop anticoagulant therapy: a cohort study. *Ann. Intern. Med.* 162 (1): 27.

27 Palareti, G., Cosmi, B., Legnani, C. et al. (2014). D-dimer to guide the duration of anticoagulation in patients with venous thromboembolism: a management study. *Blood* 124 (2): 196–203.

28 Marik, P.E. and Cavallazzi, R. (2015). Extended anticoagulant and aspirin treatment for the secondary prevention of thromboembolic disease: a systematic review and meta-analysis. *PLoS One* 10 (11): e0143252.

29 Weitz, J.I., Lensing, A.W.A., Prins, M.H. et al. (2017). Rivaroxaban or aspirin for extended treatment of venous thromboembolism. *N. Engl. J. Med.* 376 (13): 1211–1222.

30 Schulman, S., Kearon, C., Kakkar, A.K. et al. (2013). Extended use of dabigatran, warfarin, or placebo in venous thromboembolism. *N. Engl. J. Med.* 368 (8): 709–718.

31 Raskob, G., Ageno, W., Cohen, A.T. et al. (2016). Extended duration of anticoagulation with edoxaban in patients with venous thromboembolism: a post-hoc analysis of the Hokusai-VTE study. *Lancet Haematol.* 3 (5): e228–e236.

32 Agnelli, G., Buller, H.R., Cohen, A. et al. (2013). Apixaban for extended treatment of venous thromboembolism. *N. Engl. J. Med.* 368 (8): 699–708.

33 Barritt, D.W. and Jordan, S.C. (1960). Anticoagulant drugs in the treatment of pulmonary embolism. A controlled trial. *Lancet Lond Engl.* 1 (7138): 1309–1312.

34 Lagerstedt, C.I., Fagher, B.O., Olsson, C.-G. et al. (1985). Need for long-term anticoagulant treatment in symptomatic calf-vein thrombosis. *Lancet* 326 (8454): 515–518.

35 Konstantinides, S.V., Meyer, G., Becattini, C. et al. (2020). 2019 ESC Guidelines for the diagnosis and management of acute pulmonary embolism developed in collaboration with the European Respiratory Society (ERS). *Eur. Heart J.* 41 (4): 543–603.

36 Hull, R., Delmore, T., Genton, E. et al. (1979). Warfarin sodium versus low-dose heparin in the long-term treatment of venous thrombosis. *N. Engl. J. Med.* 301 (16): 855–858.

37 Hull, R.D., Raskob, G.E., Brant, R.F. et al. (1997). Relation between the time to achieve the lower limit of the APTT therapeutic range and recurrent venous thromboembolism during heparin treatment for deep vein thrombosis. *Arch. Intern. Med.* 157 (22): 2562–2568.

38 Palareti, G., Legnani, C., Cosmi, B. et al. (2005). Poor anticoagulation quality in the first 3 months after unprovoked venous thromboembolism is a risk factor for long-term recurrence. *J. Thromb. Haemost. JTH* 3 (5): 955–961.

15

Lower-Extremity Venous Stenting

Asma Khaliq[1], Sandrine Labrune[1], and Cristina Sanina[2]

[1] Department of Cardiology, Lenox Hill Heart & Vascular Institute, Donald and Barbara Zucker School of Medicine at Hofstra/Northwell Health, New York, NY, USA
[2] Division of Cardiology, Department of Medicine, Beth Israel Deaconess Medical Center, Harvard Medical School, Boston, MA, USA

Introduction

There three major type of outflow obstruction: 1) Post-thrombotic non-occlusive obstruction; 2) Post-thrombotic occlusive; 3) Non-thrombotic iliac vein lesions (May-Thurner Syndrome).

Post-thrombotic syndrome (PTS) (non-occlusive and occlusive) occur as a complication of acute deep vein thrombosis manifesting in leg pain that limits activity, edema, and leg ulcers. PTS will develop in 20–50% of patients and severe PTS, including venous ulcers in up to 10% of patients [1]. Risk of PTS is high with proximal DVT involving iliac or common femoral vein [2]. The Villalta scale has been developed, used and validated to diagnose PTS (Table 15.1) [3]. In selected patients with severe PTS endovascular treatment of chronic femoroiliocaval venous disease can be safely performed with acceptable patency result and symptoms alleviation [4].

For May-Thurnes syndrome (non-thrombotic left common iliac vein compression by right common iliac artery [Figure 15.1]), endovascular treatment is highly successful, leading to significant clinical improvement: 50% of patients has symptoms resolution, 33% experience symptoms relieve and 55% has complete healing of venous ulcers. Patency of iliac stent is 75% in 3 years. Close follow-up is mandatory to recognize the recurrence of the symptoms which can indicate stent thrombosis or re-stenosis [5, 6].

Step 1. Place the patient in the supine position for planned femoral vein access in case of iliofemoral DVT. Choose prone positioning if planning on popliteal

Endovascular Interventions: A Step-by-Step Approach, First Edition. Edited by Jose M. Wiley, Cristina Sanina, George D. Dangas, and Prakash Krishnan.
© 2023 John Wiley & Sons Ltd. Published 2023 by John Wiley & Sons Ltd.

Table 15.1 Villalta PTS Scale.

Villalta PTS scale

Assessment of:

- Five symptoms (pain, cramps, heaviness, pruritus, paresthesia) by patient self-report
- Six signs (edema, skin induration, hyperpigmentation, venous ectasia, redness, pain during calf compression) by clinician assessment

Severity of each symptom and sign is rated as 0 (absent), 1 (mild), 2 (moderate), or 3 (severe). In addition, ulcer is noted as present or absent.

Points are summed to yield the total Villalta score:

0–4:	No PTS
5–9:	Mild PTS
10–14:	Moderate PTS
≥15, or presence of ulcer	Severe PTS

Source: Adopted from Utne et al. [3].

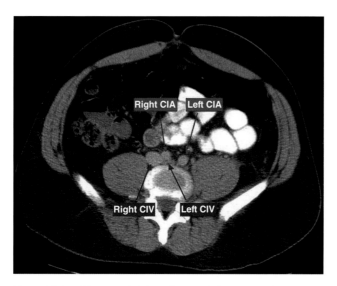

Figure 15.1 CT scan axial view showing left common iliac vein (CIV) compression by right common iliac artery (CIA). *Source:* Case courtesy of Donna D'Souza, Radiopaedia.org, rID: 4373.

vein access. The popliteal vein is located in the popliteal fossa between the popliteal artery and tibial nerve. Generally, the vein is lateral to the artery proximally in the popliteal fossa and medial to the popliteal artery distally.

TIP: Place the patient in a slight reverse Trendelenburg position. It helps dilate the vein for easier puncture.

Step 2. Anesthesia:
  Light conscious sedation is favored over general anesthesia.

Step 3. Intraprocedural use of anticoagulation.

a) Use of unfractionated heparin or bivalirudin during the procedure varies depending on the patient's pathology and the proceduralist preferences.
b) For patients with DVT, after thrombolysis, underlying occlusive venous disease might be noticed on intravascular ultrasound (IVUS).

Step 4. Use the ultrasound to identify the best femoral vein access point:
  Identify the femoral vein for planned access at the proximal or mid-thigh level. Avoid injury to the superficial femoral artery, typically anterior to the femoral vein. We recommend bilateral femoral vein access. Depending on the interventionist, the contralateral common femoral vein can be used as a secondary access point for better visualization of the confluence.

Step 5. Vascular access:
  Use a micropuncture kit. It generally includes a 21-gauge needle, a 5-Fr (sometimes 4 Fr) sheath, and a 40-cm-long 0.018-in. Cope wire. The micropuncture sheath can be upsized as needed after the guidewire is in place.
  Applying the Seldinger technique: Over a sterile field, get access with a 21-gauge needle under ultrasound guidance. Place Cope wire through needle. Remove the needle over the Cope wire and replace with a micropuncture sheath. Remove the guidewire and advance the glide wire through the 5 Fr sheath under fluoroscopy. Ensure under fluoroscopy that the glide wire is through the femoral vein with sufficient purchase (high up enough) before introducing the sheath. Lesions that are not 100% obstructed allow the glide wire and glide catheter to go through easily. In presence of occlusion, a stiff glide wire with a 0.035-in. support catheter may be needed. Further progress into the occlusion is made with the tip of the glide wire with straight or angled catheter support.

Step 6. Sheath upgrade:
  Once access is satisfactory, switch the wire to a stiff 0.035 supra core wire (Figure 15.2) and exchange to a 9 or 10 Fr sheath. The supra core is a supportive

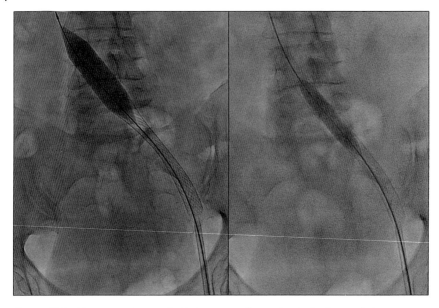

Figure 15.2 Venogram. Access site left common femoral vein. Exchange 4 Fr or 5 Fr micro puncture catheter over 0.035″ supra core wire placed in IVC to 9 Fr or 10 Fr sheath.

wire with a soft atraumatic tip with great steering and facilitates catheter placement for diagnostic and contralateral approach interventions.

Step 7. Imaging:

a) After vascular access is established, antegrade venography under fluoroscopy is performed to identify the anatomic landmarks and determine the degree, length, and site of obstruction, and the presence of collateral vessels.
   i) Ipsilateral injection 10 ml/s–15 ml for 900 PSI is done on AP position under DSA.
   ii) Contrast venography is poorly sensitive to iliac vein obstruction.
b) Following the venogram, use of IVUS (IVUS is 10 Fr compatible) is strongly encouraged to make an accurate diagnosis and to aid in treatment strategy for stent deployment and landing zone for instance.
   i) IVUS aids in mapping the venous system from the femoral vein to the inferior vena cava (IVC): common femoral vein, external iliac vein, common iliac vein, and IVC.
   ii) A decrease in lumen size by more than 50% suggests obstruction that requires close evaluation and/or intervention.

Step 8. Once the area of venous stenosis/obstruction is identified:

a) After crossing the lesion with a guidewire, dilatation can be done before (pre-dilatation) or after stent deployment, at the discretion of the proceduralist.
   i) **Tip:** To monitor the progress of the recanalization, obtain 45° or 60° oblique projections to ensure that the glide wire initially follows the curve of the sacrum and then turns anterior to the spine.
   ii) Predilate using a 6–8 mm balloon, up to 4 atm, for an inflation time of 30 seconds to one minute.
   iii) Avoid using large balloons for predilation or predilating to the desired diameter.

Step 9. Once the identified lesion is dilated, determine the size of the stent.

a) Use IVUS intraprocedurally to estimate best stent sizing:
   i) Measure the diameter and length of the vessel proximal and distal to the desired landing zone.
   ii) TIP: If the contralateral iliac vein is free of disease, the diameter of the vessel (by IVUS or preprocedural imaging) can be used for sizing reference.
   iii) Oversizing the stent by up to 4 mm (2–4 mm) for the anatomic location is recommended to compensate for the potential recoil of the recanalized vessel.

Step 10. Stent deployment:

a) Currently, FDA approved options for venous stenting include stainless steel and nitinol stents, as well as covered stent-graft. The Wallstent; Closed (8–24 mm/20–90 mm), Vici Veniti by Boston Scientific; Closed (12–16 mm/60–120 mm), Bard Venovo; Open (10–20 mm/40–60 mm).
b) Stents shouldn't be used more distally to the inguinal ligament due to the risk of stent fracture from hip flexion.
c) The Wallstent is a closed (8–24 mm/20–90 mm), self-expanding stainless steel stent with great strength and flexibility.
   i) It is weakest at the end and foreshortening makes precise placement difficult.
d) Start beyond the lesion up to below the lesion. It is important that both ends of the stent land in normal looking tissue.
   i) For nonthrombotic lesions, like NIVL for instance, start the deployment, 2–3 cm into the IVC. A deployment over 3 cm risks obstructing flow to the contralateral iliac vein.
   ii) TIP: The Wallstent is retrievable up to a certain point before complete deployment, a helpful feature for when the location of the stent is not optimal.

(a)   (b)

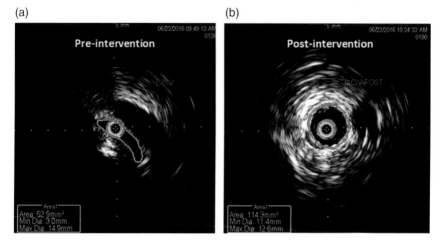

Figure 15.3 Postdeployment series of Wallstent dilatation placed in left iliac vein.

    iii) When using multiple stents, ensure 3–5 cm overlap **(some say 2–3 cm)** between these stents.
    iv) Optimal stent diameters after recoil:
        1) 20 mm for the IVC
        2) 16–18 mm for the common iliac vein
        3) 14–16 mm for the external iliac vein
        4) 12–14 mm for the common femoral vein
  e) Postdeployment dilatation:
      i) This step is recommended even if the stent appears fully extended.
     ii) Prevent foreshortening of the Wallstent by ballooning the side closest to the lesions (Figure 15.3). Stent will foreshorten as it gains in diameter. Therefore, if the stent is only placed in the lesion area (and not from normal tissue to normal tissue), over time that stent will no longer be covering the area of stenosis.
    iii) Perform balloon angioplasty using high-pressure, large-diameter balloons (12–20 mm × 4–6 cm) with prolonged inflation time (>30 seconds up to 1 minute) to ensure adequate wall apposition.

Step 11. Poststenting evaluation:

IVUS is favored over multiplane venography to ensure there is no residual obstruction, especially distally, incomplete dilatation, or improper stent apposition (Figure 15.4). When any residual obstruction or lesion is seen, further intervention with repeat angioplasty is required.

(a)   (b)

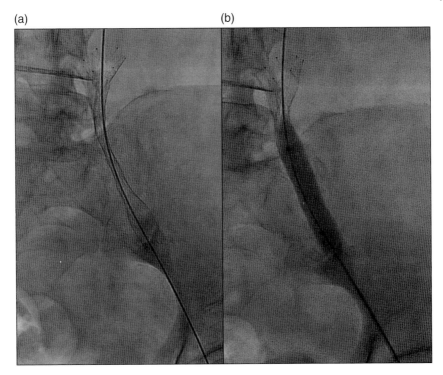

Figure 15.4 IVUS guided venous stenting, left iliac vein. (a) Pre-intervention left iliac vein stenosis by IVUS. (b) Post-intervention: optimal stent apposition and left iliac vein stenosis resolution by IVUS.

Step 12. Sheath care:

Remove the sheath after applying the "Figure of 8 or 3-Way Stop-Cock" suture technique and apply light pressure until homeostasis is achieved.

Follow-Up

No bed rest needed poststenting. Patient expected to have severe back discomfort for up to one week postprocedurally. Start AC (warfarin or rivaroxaban) night of day of intervention (up to one year). Routine follow-up usually occurs 1, 3, 9, and 18 months after intervention. If patient returns symptomatic (leg swelling, pelvic edema, persistent leg pain, varicose veins, etc.) repeat venogram/IVUS.

References

1 Kahn, S.R., Comerota, A.J., Cushman, M. et al. (2014). American Heart Association Council on Peripheral Vascular Disease, Council on Clinical Cardiology, and Council on Cardiovascular and Stroke Nursing. The postthrombotic syndrome: evidence-based prevention, diagnosis, and treatment strategies: a scientific statement from the American Heart Association. *Circulation*. 130 (18): 1636–1661.

2 Kahn, S.R. (2016). The post-thrombotic syndrome. *Hematology Am. Soc. Hematol. Educ. Program*. 2016 (1): 413–418.

3 Utne, K.K., Ghanima, W., Foyn, S. et al. (2016). Development and validation of a tool for patient reporting of symptoms and signs of the post-thrombotic syndrome. *Thromb. Haemost.* 115 (2): 361–367.

4 Wahlgren, C.-M., Wahlberg, E., and Olofsson, P. (2010). Endovascular Treatment in Postthrombotic Syndrome. *Vascular and Endovascular Surgery*. 44 (5): 356–360.

5 Danza, R., Navarro, T., and Baldizan, J. (1991). Reconstructive surgery in chronic venous obstruction of the lower limbs. *J. Cardiovasc. Surg.* 32: 98–103.

6 Neglen, P. and Raju, S. (2002). Intravascular ultrasound scan evaluation of the obstructed vein. *J. Vasc. Surg.* 35: 694–700.

16

Intervention for Pulmonary Embolism

Seth I. Sokol[1], Wissam A. Jaber[2], and Yosef Golowa[3]

[1] Division of Cardiovascular Diseases, Albert Einstein College of Medicine-Jacobi Medical Center, Bronx, NY, USA
[2] Division of Cardiology, Emory University Hospital, Atlanta, GA, USA
[3] Department of Radiology, Albert Einstein College of Medicine-Montefiore Medical Center, Bronx, NY, USA

Introduction

Sub-massive or massive, central or saddle pulmonary embolism (PE) is a severe condition that can cause cardiogenic shock, death or chronic pulmonary hypertension. Systemic thrombolysis with rt-PA or alteplase (approved by FDA) is only used in hemodynamically unstable and peri-code/ code patients. Catheter – directed therapies have been emerging as attractive option and warrant optimal angiographic result, reduction in RV/LV ration and decrease in pulmonary hypertension.

Pulmonary Angiography

Despite the advent of CTA, pulmonary angiography retains an important role in diagnosis and treatment of PE especially to selectively guide interventional treatment [1].

Vascular Access

Access can be obtained in the common femoral vein, brachial vein, or internal jugular vein using ultrasound guidance and a micro-puncture needle kit.

Endovascular Interventions: A Step-by-Step Approach, First Edition. Edited by Jose M. Wiley, Cristina Sanina, George D. Dangas, and Prakash Krishnan.
© 2023 John Wiley & Sons Ltd. Published 2023 by John Wiley & Sons Ltd.

Injection and X-Ray Detector Positioning

A balloon-tipped catheter with multiple sideholes (for example, Arrow® Berman™ catheter, Teleflex, Morrisville, NC, USA) is advanced into the main pulmonary artery. Right atrial, ventricular, and pulmonary artery pressures can be measured.

Note: Arrow Berman catheter does not have an endhole and therefore cannot be used for wire exchanges.
Alternative: 5 or 6 Fr angled Pigtail catheter delivered over a 0.035 J-tip or angled tip wire.

For 9 in. detectors, given the limited field, a nonselective angiogram in the main PA may not include the peripheral pulmonary vasculature.

Tip: The table should be raised as high as possible and flat panel positioned as close to patient as possible to maximize the amount of lung imaged.

A more selective angiogram of the right and left pulmonary arteries can be performed to assess the entire lung field. RAO 20° for right PA and LAO 20° for left PA. Each injection should be with 30–40 ml of dye given over two seconds ("15 for 30 or 20 for 40").For 12 in. or greater detectors, position catheter tip in the trunk of the main pulmonary artery and inject 40 ml of dye over two seconds ("20 for 40"). Further selective imaging can then be done if needed.

Notes: (i) A PA systolic pressure greater than 80 mmHg is a contraindication to pulmonary angiography with a power injector. (ii) The presence of a left bundle branch block may require a temporary pacing wire given the risk of inducing complete heart block with right heart catheter manipulation.

Catheter-Directed Thrombolysis

EKOS™ Catheter-Directed Thrombolysis

The EkoSonic (BTG, London, England) endovascular system is FDA approved for the treatment of pulmonary embolism (Figure 16.1). The device allows for infusion of thrombolytics in the pulmonary arteries while delivering ultrasound energy waves to increase the dispersion of the drug within the thrombus.

The infusion catheter is 5.4 Fr and multi-lumen including a coolant lumen allowing for guidewire insertion for catheter delivery, injection of contrast (maximum of 200 PSI) and continuous infusion of saline to cool the ultrasonic core. A drug delivery lumen with perforated holes allows for delivery of drug along and around the chosen treatment length zone (Figure 16.2a,b).

Note: Drug delivery lumens are closed to distal end of infusion treatment zone.

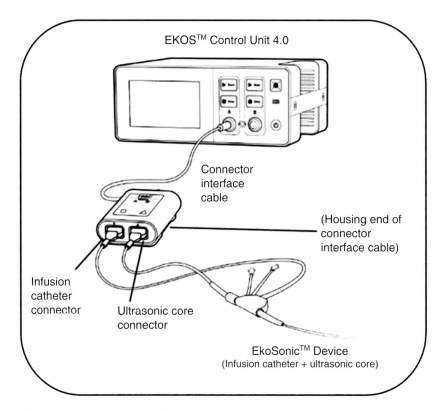

EKOS™ Control Unit 4.0

Connector interface cable

(Housing end of connector interface cable)

Infusion catheter connector

Ultrasonic core connector

EkoSonic™ Device
(Infusion catheter + ultrasonic core)

Figure 16.1 Second-generation device consists of a control unit to deliver power to up to two catheters (first generation only allowed for one catheter) with a user interface, and a connector interface cable that connects the infusion catheter and ultrasonic core to the control unit. *Source:* With permission from BTG.

Preparation of System

Step 1. Two infusion pumps should be prepared; one for delivery of coolant (heparinized saline) and the other for drug.

Step 2. After selecting a catheter based on treatment zone length (usually a 12 cm active ultrasound core length on a 106 cm or 135 cm catheter) stopcocks are attached to luers labeled "Coolant" and "Drug" and flushed with heparinized saline. Fluid should be seen exiting the catheter holes along the treatment zone when injecting the drug port (Figure 16.3).

Tips: (i) A towel should be wrapped around the electrical connector plugs to prevent contact with fluids. (ii) Priming volume of coolant lumen is 1.9 cc's.

(a)

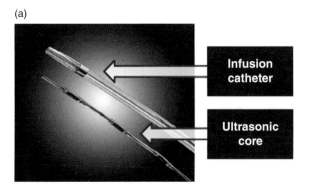

(b)

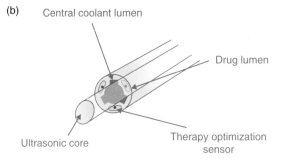

Figure 16.2   (a) Infusion catheter tip and ultrasonic core. (b) Cross-section of multi-lumen infusion catheter. *Source:* With permission from BTG.

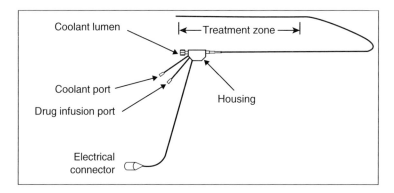

Figure 16.3   EKOS infusion catheter. *Source:* With permission from BTG.

Access

The EKOS catheter requires placement of one or two 6 Fr sheaths depending on whether treatment of one or both lungs is required. Options include single or dual access in the common femoral (double puncture in tandem) or use of any of the following sites as stand-alone or as a second access for double lung treatment: common femoral vein, brachial/basilic veins, or internal jugular vein.

Step 1. A 4, 5 or 6 Fr JR4 catheter is advanced over a 0.35 in. 260 cm J-tipped or angled tip wire into the right or left pulmonary artery. The tip of the wire should be placed in a distal branch pulmonary artery.

Tip: Typically, the infusion catheter can be advanced on its own over a guidewire that has been already positioned in the pulmonary artery (see below) without the need for a long sheath or guide. A long sheath can be helpful to provide more support for catheter delivery when needed.

Safety Tip: An angled glide wire can be used but caution should be taken to avoid buckling of the wire or pushing through resistance to avoid perforation. A loop at the tip of the wire is helpful and likely protective and should be advanced down an artery without any resistance.

Step 2. The JR4 catheter is then removed with care to maintain wire position and exchanged out for the EKOS endhole catheter. Typically, a 12 cm treatment length × 106 total length is used.

Tip: If the infusion catheter cannot be advanced through the RV and PA due to angle and/or poor support, the JR4 can be used to exchange for a stiffer wire or a long sheath guide can be positioned in or near the right atrium and used for better support.

Step 3. Once infusion catheter is delivered (should be in distal branch – Figure 16.4), the wire is removed and blood is aspirated back to remove bubbles and then flushed with heparinized saline. Via the drug delivery port, a priming bolus or greater of tpa can be given if desired

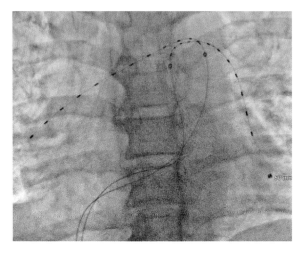

Figure 16.4 Appropriate final catheter positions.

Tip: A minimum of 0.8 cc for the 106 cm and 1.0 cc for the 135 cm length catheter of tpa is needed for priming the catheter.

Safety Tip: Blood should never be drawn back into the drug delivery lumen.

Step 4. The inner ultrasonic core is carefully removed from its packaging and moistened with heparinized saline. It is then inserted and advanced through the infusion catheters main coolant lumen (not port) and once fully advanced the luer connectors on the catheter and ultrasound core are secured together.

Tip: Do not kink ultrasound core – if any kinking occurs will need to discard and open new ultrasonic core.

The same is repeated for the second lung if desired. A completion stored fluoro or cine should be performed to document final catheter placement location (Figure 16.4).

Infusion of tpa is then initiated. Dosing regimens of tpa and heparin can be based on the ULTIMA [2], SEATLE II [3], or Optalyse PE [4] studies. The author uses alteplase 1 mg/h per lung and typically infuses 300–400 units of heparin via each access sheath to maintain patency while avoiding systemic therapeutic levels (PTT < 45) which may raise the risk of bleeding.

Note: Other standard infusion catheters can be used that do not provide ultrasound. These include the UniFuse and the Craig–McNamara catheters. They are delivered in the same fashion as the EKOS infusion catheter. No prospective trials have been reported comparing EKOS to standard CDT. The SUNSET PE trial is currently investigating that question.

Mechanical Disruption

Catheter Fragmentation of Clot

The most common technique is to utilize a pigtail catheter and place it within the clot and simply rotate the catheter vigorously as to fragment the thrombus. Angioplasty balloon maceration can also be used to disrupt and fragment the clot.

Tip: These techniques only cause fragmentation and disruption and likely distal embolization. The concept is that there is more surface area in the distal branches of the pulmonary artery, and by sending fragments to these branches, resistance in the pulmonary arteries may improve.

Large Catheter Aspiration

FlowTriever™

The FlowTriever (Inari Medical, Irvine, CA, USA) thrombus aspiration system consists of a 20 Fr, 95 cm catheter (F20, a in Figure 16.5), with a hemostatic valve (b),

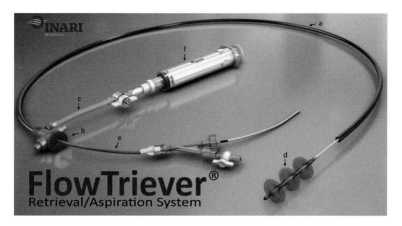

Figure 16.5 FlowTriever thrombus aspiration system. *Source:* INARI Medicals.

and a large-bore side port for aspiration (c). The optional self-deploying nitinol disks (d) come in three sizes (between 6 and 18 mm), and are mounted on a catheter (e) designed to be advanced inside the F20 to engage the thrombus in the blood vessel.

A new 16 Fr catheter (F16) is available if more distal thrombi in smaller vessels need to be accessed, and can be intussuscepted inside the F20 if needed. The system received FDA approval for the treatment of acute PE in 2018 based on the FLARE trial [5], a single-arm multicenter prospective study of 106 patients with acute PE and right ventricle to left ventricle ratio of >0.9 by CT scan treated with the FlowTriever catheter. The FLARE trial showed an improvement in this ratio from baseline to 48 hours after the procedure, with no major device-related complications.

Access

Step 1. The procedure is usually performed under conscious sedation using a femoral approach (right preferred). Ultrasound-guided access is advised to reduce vascular complications and to exclude femoral/iliac thrombus at the access site. After serial dilation over a stiff wire, a 22 Fr sheath (for example DrySeal, Gore, Newark, DE, USA) is placed in the femoral vein. All patients should be anticoagulated once access in securely obtained.

Step 2. Using a balloon-tipped catheter, a right heart catheterization is performed with documentation of right atrial and PA pressures and cardiac output. These measurements can be repeated at the end of the procedure to document any changes attributable to the treatment.

Safety Tip: The tricuspid valve should be crossed using a balloon-tipped catheter to avoid entrapment under a tricuspid valve cord to avoid valve damage during advancement of the F20 (Figure 16.6).

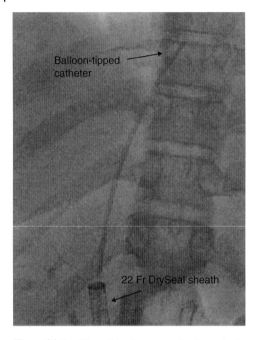

Figure 16.6 Tricuspid valve crossed using a balloon-tipped catheter to avoid entrapment under a tricuspid valve cord.

Step 3. Once the balloon catheter is in the PA and measurements are made, a long 0.035 in. wire is used to exchange the balloon catheter to a diagnostic catheter (for example a multipurpose or pigtail cardiac catheter) to direct the wire into the desired PA branch. A PA angiogram is performed to define the location of the obstructive thrombi (Figure 16.7); with the presence of a hemodynamically significant PE, a manual injection is sufficient.

Step 4. Once the target thrombus is identified (typically in the main left or right, lower interlobar, or right middle lobar branch), a guidewire is advanced distally. A multipurpose or a JR4 catheter is helpful in directing the guidewire in the desired branch. Injection of a small amount of contrast in the distal vessel helps ensure the catheter is in a reasonably sized artery to accommodate an exchange length wire, and document that the catheter has crossed the obstructed branch (Figure 16.8).

Safety Tip: Although helpful in crossing obstructive thrombi, hydrophilic wires should be used extremely carefully – if at all – in the distal vessels to avoid perforations.

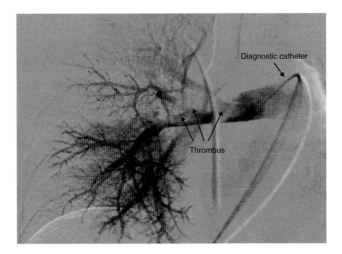

Figure 16.7 PA angiogram defining location of proximal thrombus.

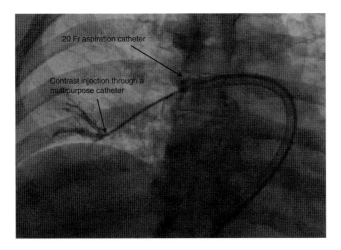

Figure 16.8 Contrast injection through the multipurpose catheter.

Step 5. Over a supportive exchange length wire, the F20 with its dilator are advanced until they engage the thrombus. The dilator is then removed while the wire remains in place, and the aspiration syringe is attached to the side port.

Tip: For an effective aspiration, the F20 tip has to engage the thrombus first or be just in front of it. This also minimizes blood loss by creating a dry suctioning.

Step 6. While suction is applied, and in the absence of blood return, the authors typically wait at least 30 seconds to give time to part of the thrombus to conform inside the distal tip of the catheter. If the syringe fills, it is emptied and blood examined for thrombi. The F20 is then repositioned in preparation for more aspiration. If there is no blood return, the whole catheter is withdrawn over the wire while under suction and flushed outside the body, usually yielding part of the pulmonary embolus (examples in Figure 16.9.)

Step 7. To redirect to a different branch or to the other lung, the diagnostic catheter is reintroduced over the wire and the above steps are repeated. If aspiration is unsuccessful at removing thrombi, especially when the latter are impacted in the distal vessels, the self-deploying disks can be advanced over the wire inside the F20 and unsheathed in the distal vessel (Figure 16.10).

Once deployed, they are withdrawn into the F20 while syringe aspiration is activated.

Tip: Merely withdrawing the disks without negative suctioning is unlikely to be effective in thrombus removal.

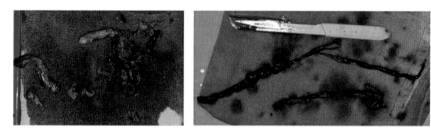

Figure 16.9 Thrombi extracted via aspiration through the F20.

(a)   (b)

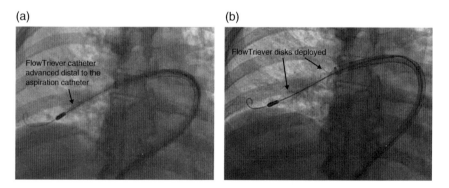

Figure 16.10 Positioning (a) and deployment (b) of FlowTriever catheter and disks.

Notes: The endpoint of the aspiration process is poorly defined. The authors typically terminate the procedure when one or more of the following occurs: (i) patient significantly feels better with improvement in saturation and/ or heart rate; (ii) significant thrombus has been removed with evidence of better perfusion on angiography; (iii) significant improvement in PA pressure and/or cardiac output has been achieved; and (iv) no thrombi are being removed despite multiple passes, typically seen in the more chronic emboli.

Step 8. Hemostasis can be achieved either with a mattress or figure-of-8 suture, or with a closure device (Proglide) deployed prior to insertion of the large sheath.

Note: Large catheter aspiration is attractive for patients with high-risk PE with contraindication to thrombolysis and for patients with intermediate-risk PE at risk for deterioration, especially when thrombolytic use is to be avoided. Patients stabilized with this procedure may avoid ICU stay. Potential complications include those of vascular access, tricuspid valve or cardiac injury, PA perforation/hemorrhage, or hemodynamic/pulmonary deterioration related to distal embolization of saddle or intracardiac thrombi.

Penumbra

The Penumbra's Indigo® system (Penumbra Inc., Alameda, CA, USA) does not have a specific approval for use in the pulmonary arteries, but it is FDA approved for removal of thrombus in the peripheral venous and arterial system. The thrombectomy catheters suction by continuous vacuum generated aspiration through its Penumbra Engine™ (Penumbra Inc., Alameda, CA, USA) aspiration source.

For the purpose of thrombectomy for proximal pulmonary emboli, the largest catheter CAT8 (Continuous Aspiration Mechanical Thrombectomy Catheter 8) should be used. The CAT8 is available in three shapes: Straight (85 cm), Torq (85 cm), and XTorq (115 cm). The author prefers the XTorq shape (115 cm), given length and ability for circumferential aspiration. A #8 separator is needed to clear the lumen of the aspiration catheter during active suction.

Step 1. Obtain ultrasound-guided venous access (femoral or jugular) using standard technique. A 65 or 90 cm 8 Fr sheath guide (Terumo Pinnacle® Destination®, TERUMO Medical Corporation, Somerset, NJ, USA), or long sheath should be advanced over a wire (0.035 angled or J-tip wire) into the RA or proximal portion of the targeted pulmonary artery.

Tips: (i) A 90 cm length sheath cannot be used if the CAT8 straight (85 cm) or CAT8 Torq (85 cm) is used due to length mismatch. (ii) If using a Cook Flexor® sheath (Cook Medical LLC, Bloomington, IN, USA), with a Check-Flo valve a

10 Fr is required to accommodate the CAT8. (iii) A 6 Fr JR4 catheter can be telescoped through the sheath guide or long sheath to help steer the guidewire into the pulmonary artery.

Step 2. Once access is obtained, the patient is heparinized (80–100 U/kg bolus) to an ACT ≥250.

Step 3. The packaging of the aspiration catheter and its lumen and separator are flushed with heparinized saline. The catheter is inserted through a rotating hemostasis valve on the guide sheath or through the valve of the sheath using the peelable introducer sheath on the aspiration catheter. Once inserted the peelable sheath is removed from the aspiration catheter.

Tip: The peelable sheath can be kept on the catheter in the event the catheter needs to be removed from the sheath and then reinserted.

Step 4. The aspiration catheter is advanced over the wire into the targeted segment in the pulmonary artery and positioned immediately proximal to the thrombus. The guidewire is then removed. Contrast can be injected through the aspiration catheter to obtain a selective pulmonary angiogram to visualize thrombus locations. If not contraindicated, a small bolus of tpa (2–5 mg) can also be injected through the aspiration catheter.

Step 5. Aspiration tubing is then attached to the aspiration pump and turned on. The valve on the aspiration tubing should be in the OFF position. Gauge should read −20 mmHg or greater.

Step 6. The aspiration catheter is advanced and embedded in the thrombus. A #8 separator is then inserted through the rotating hemostasis valve into the aspiration catheter. The aspiration tubing is connected to the side port of the rotating hemostasis valve. The valve on the aspiration tubing is switched to ON to begin aspiration, and the separator is advanced and retracted during active suction. The aspiration catheter can be rotated to engage additional thrombus.

Safety Tips: (i) Never retract, advance, or torque the catheter or separator against resistance as this could lead to vessel damage and perforation. (ii) The separator should not be used as a guidewire to advance the catheter.

Step 7. To stop aspiration the aspiration tubing valve is switched to the OFF position and then the pump can be turned OFF. The separator is removed. A volume of 5–10 ml of blood should be aspirated from the catheter and once the catheter is cleared, it can be used to hand inject contrast. If further treatment of smaller distal branches (vessel size 2–3 mm) is needed, the CAT3 device can be used by telescoping through the existing sheath or CAT8 device.

Safety Tip: During active aspiration a nurse or technician should pay close attention to the amount and speed of blood removal into container. This should be continuously verbalized to the operator. When the aspiration catheter is engaged in thrombus, blood is seen slowly dripping out into the canister. If flow stops completely despite use of the separator, the catheter should be withdrawn and flushed to remove trapped thrombus. If blood flow is more rapid and continuous, this is indicative that clot is not being engaged or removed and flow should be either interrupted or the catheter repositioned to avoid excessive blood loss. If there is substantial aspiration of blood as the procedure warrants, consideration can be made to replete with a packed red blood cell transfusion.

AngioVac

The AngioVac® system (Angiodynamic, Latham, NY, USA) is a large-bore suction thrombectomy device indicated for removal of fresh, soft thrombi or emboli during extracorporeal bypass. The system utilizes a 22 French coil reinforced aspiration cannula with an expandable funnel tip that can engage and aspirate large thrombi. Aspiration is achieved by attaching the cannula to a cardiopulmonary bypass circuit, where the blood is filtered and then is then returned to the patient via a large-bore return cannula via a second central venous access (Figure 16.11).

It currently is available in straight, and 20° configurations with a balloon-actuated expandable funnel (generation 2) (Figure 16.12a) as well as a configuration (generation 3) (Figure 16.12b) which allows up to 180° angulation of the catheter by unsheathing the distal end of the cannula. The funnel on third-generation device is expanded by nitinol struts in the leaflets and is deployed by unsheathing the funnel.

Large thrombus in the setting of pulmonary embolism may be amenable to removal utilizing the AngioVac system [6, 7]. The AngioVac also shows promise in the treatment of clot-in-transit in the right atrium/ventricle [8]. It can also be utilized effectively for debulking large infected right heart vegetations to prevent septic pulmonary embolism [9, 10].

Patient Selection and Central Venous Access

As this device requires large-bore sheath and cannula access into central veins, documentation of patency of two suitable accesses should be ascertained, including evaluation of both internal jugular veins and both common femoral veins. There should be no absolute contraindication to anticoagulation. Patients with heparin allergies can be anticoagulated with argatroban or bivalirudin. Right heart vegetation procedures are often facilitated in conjunction with real-time transesophageal echocardiography (TEE) guidance, necessitating anesthesia

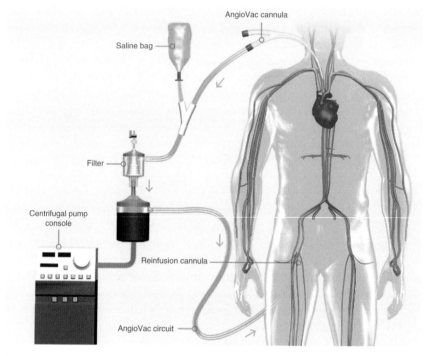

Figure 16.11 AngioVac system utilizes a large intravascular cannula attached to a cardiopulmonary bypass circuit where blood is filtered and then returned to patient. *Source:* Image courtesy of AngioDynamics, Inc. and its affiliates.

(a)   (b)

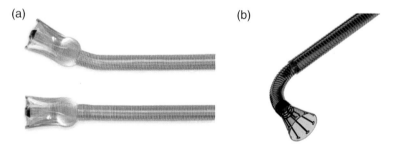

Figure 16.12 (a) Generation 2 device with balloon-actuated funnel, straight and 20° fixed angulation. Source: Courtesy of AngioDynamics, Inc. (b) Generation 3 device with funnel expanded by nitinol struts and flexible cannula up to 180° angulation. *Source:* Courtesy of AngioDynamics, Inc.

services, and an operator of the echocardiography imaging equipment. Intracardiac echocardiography (ICE) has also been used to facilitate right heart vegetation removal [11], which may obviate the need for general anesthesia. Clot-in-transit embolectomy procedures can be performed with intraprocedural transthoracic echocardiography (TTE) monitoring, as general anesthesia may not be desirable in patients with pulmonary embolus.

AngioVac Circuit Setup and Thrombus Aspiration

Step 1. Venous access should be obtained in two central veins (internal jugular vein or common femoral veins). Ultrasound guidance is recommended for access to avoid inadvertent arterial injury before large-bore sheath placement and anticoagulation.

Tip: The preclose technique can be performed after obtaining access, before dilating to larger French size at the venous access sites by placing a purse-string suture at each access site or placing a single Perclose ProGlide (Abbott, Santa Clara, CA, USA) suture at this time if desired.

Step 2. Intravenous anticoagulant bolus can be administered at this point before placement of reinfusion cannula to prevent thrombus from forming in the cannula (a minimum target of ACT of 300 is desired while blood is in the circuit).

Step 3. Serial dilatation is then performed at each venous access site, respectively, 16 or 18 Fr reinfusion cannula is placed at one site, and a 26 Fr DrySeal sheath (W.L. Gore, Flagstaff, AZ, USA) is placed at the site desired for aspiration.

Step 4. The circuit is opened in the sterile field, and the Y-circuit hub is connected to the female connector, closing the circuit of the operator's side (Figure 16.13a). A Tuohy-Borst adaptor is inserted into the red Tuohy on the Y-adapter; both are tightened to finger tight (Figure 16.13b). An adequate amount of sterile circuit tubing is left on the field, and the remainder of the circuit is passed off to perfusionist for circuit assembly (perfusion circuit assembly is not included in this description).

Step 5. After the circuit is primed, clamps are placed on the ends of the tubing, marked by a blue line and red line, respectively, ensuring the circuit remains primed (Figure 16.13c). The two ends are then separated again. A wet-to-wet connection is made at the reinfusion cannula, ensuring there is no air in the tubing.

Tip: A stopcock and a 60 cc syringe can be used to aspirate any residual air from the return tubing.

The Y-adaptor end is connected to the AngioVac cannula (Figure 16.13d), the clamp is removed, and the cannula is then primed with saline. The Tuohy insert is removed, and the obturator is inserted until it is entirely through the distal end of AngioVac cannula (Figure 16.13e). The clamp is removed and cannula flushed. The AngioVac cannula can then be advanced through the DrySeal sheath over a wire to its desired location, and the obturator is then removed.

(a)

(b)

(c)

(d)

(e)

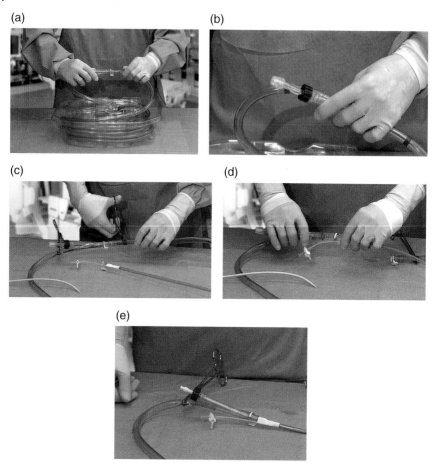

Figure 16.13 (a–e) AngioVac circuit assembly. *Source:* Courtesy of AngioDynamics, Inc.

Tip: If the AngioVac does not need significant intravascular manipulation, the cannula can be directly advanced through the DrySeal sheath without the obturator, taking care not to damage the leaflets as it enters the hub. The cannula can then be unsheathed to avoid advancing it into the vessel wall.

Step 6. With the second-generation AngioVac device, an inflator is used to distend a balloon which deploys funnel. The balloon should not be inflated more than 2 mmHg as it may rupture. With the third-generation AngioVac device, the funnel is deployed by unsheathing the end of the cannula.

Tip: With the second-generation device, if the balloon ruptures, the leaflets of the cannula may not open properly, limiting flows.

Step 7. All clamps are removed, and flow is initiated and optimized to approximately 3–4l/min.

Step 8. AngioVac cannula is then advanced to engage the thrombus.

AngioVac for Pulmonary Embolus

AngioVac can engage and remove large thrombus and may be a useful tool in the treatment of large central pulmonary embolus, especially when the use of lytics may be contraindicated. Note, however, the use of AngioVac in the pulmonary arteries constitutes off label use of the device.Because of the size and rigidity of the current iteration of the cannula, manipulating through the right heart into the pulmonary arteries may prove challenging. Also, the cannula cannot be advanced past the main pulmonary arteries and may be less effective in the treatment of isolated peripheral segmental thrombus. Caution must be taken when manipulating the cannula across the tricuspid valvular apparatus during catheter placement to avoid valvular injury. When crossing the tricuspid valve, care must be taken to avoid hooking chordae tendineae of the valve. This can be achieved by using an inflated Swan–Ganz balloon catheter or a formed pigtail catheter with a tip deflecting wire to cross the valve into the right ventricle/pulmonary outflow tract. This can then be exchanged for a stiff wire, i.e. a super-stiff Amplatz wire or a Lundquist wire, to facilitate the delivery of the AngioVac cannula to the

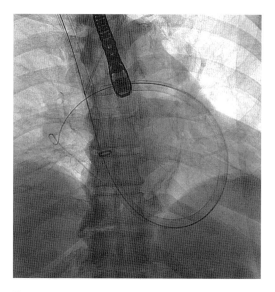

Figure 16.14 AngioVac cannula advanced to the right pulmonary artery from a right internal jugular approach. The wire was left in place to maintain position.

pulmonary artery. The cannula is advanced with the obturator to the pulmonary artery, central to the clot. The obturator is removed, the funnel expanded, and flow is then initiated before the thrombus in engaged.

Tip: It may be easier to deliver the AngioVac to the right pulmonary artery when using a right internal jugular venous approach (Figure 16.14), whereas the left pulmonary artery may be more amenable from a right femoral venous approach.

AngioVac for Clot-in-Transit

In the setting of pulmonary embolism with clot-in-transit, it may be advantageous to forgo general anesthesia if possible. Anesthesia induction can cause alterations in patient hemodynamics, which in the setting of massive pulmonary embolism may worsen clinical status [12, 13] or possibly precipitate further migration of atrial clot to the pulmonary arteries. The AngioVac procedure in this setting can be performed utilizing only local anesthesia using TTE or intravascular US (IVUS) to confirm successful removal of the thrombus.

During access and sheath placement, care should be taken to avoid wires entering the heart to prevent dislodgement of the atrial clot. Bilateral femoral vein approach would facilitate this.

Inferior vena cava venography can be performed before advancing the large cannula to exclude caval thrombus which may become dislodged.

Flow should be optimized in the inferior vena cava, and the cannula then advanced into the right atrium to engage the thrombus (Figure 16.15a).

If the flow stops in the circuit, it may be due to large thrombus obstructing the lumen (Figure 16.15b). Waiting for a few minutes "on pump" may sometimes allow the clot to fragment or conform to the cannula and pass. Increasing the RPM on the pump can also facilitate passage of clot. Another maneuver is to kink or clamp the circuit tubing and then quickly release, which causes an abrupt suction on the clot which may help it fragment and pass. If these maneuvers fail, the cannula with clot can be removed while on the pump. Placement of an IVC filter above the cannula can ensure that large clot does not dislodge during removal (Figure 16.15c–e).

AngioVac for Right Heart Vegetation

Patient Selection and Approach

Mobile vegetations which appear pedunculated are more likely to be successfully removed via suction thrombectomy, whereas firm, chronic sessile clot may prove more difficult.

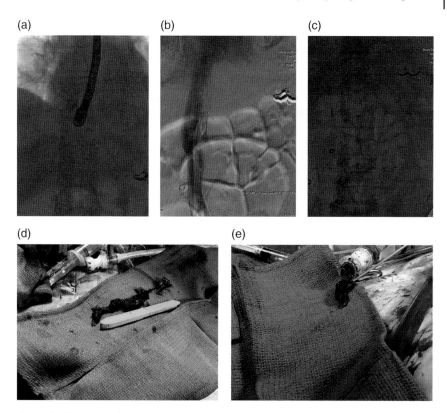

Figure 16.15 (a–e) Clot-in-transit is generally mobile and can be engaged by advancing into right atrium while on pump (a). With large clot burden, the clot could get stuck at the tip of the cannula which can have this "ice cream cone" appearance (b). If the cannula cannot be cleared, a filter can be placed above cannula before removal to prevent dislodgement (c). Most of the clot in this case was able to be removed (d), however, much of it got stuck in the valve of the sheath (e).

If the vegetation is originating from the septal leaflet of the tricuspid valve, the septal side of the right atrium, or a catheter or Pacemaker/AICD lead, a femoral venous approach for the aspiration cannula may be advantageous. For anterior or posterior tricuspid valve leaflet vegetations, the anatomy favors an internal jugular venous approach.

Technique

It may be challenging to engage vegetations with generation 2 AngioVac, straight or 20° angled cannulas. The tip of the cannula can be redirected by using a large gooseneck snare positioned between the balloon and the funnel leaflets to direct the AngioVac cannula toward the thrombus (Figure 16.16a). Alternatively, a

(a)   (b)   (c)

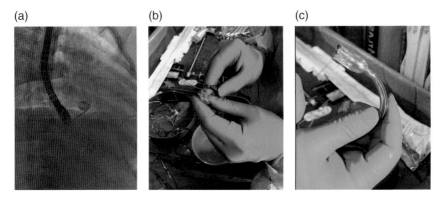

Figure 16.16 (a–c) When using generation 2 device for right heart vegetations it can be helpful to create angulations on the cannula. This can be done using a snare to angle the cannula (a), or placing a suture in one of the leaflets (b, c).

90 cm prolene suture can be tied to the inferior most leaflet of the cannula which the operator can use to angle cannula outside the sheath alongside the cannula (Figure 16.16b,c). With the third-generation device, as the distal part of the cannula is unsheathed, the cannula can make up to a 180° angulation.

After angulating toward the vegetation, the funnel is then rotated toward the target with a sweeping motion by twisting the entire cannula. Intraprocedural TEE or ICE can be used real-time to confirm the orientation of cannula to the vegetation and successful removal.

References

1 Kasper, W., Konstantinides, S., Geibel, A. et al. (1997). Management strategies and determinants of outcome in acute major pulmonary embolism: results of a multicenter registry. *Journal of the American College of Cardiology* 30: 1165–1171.

2 Kucher, N., Boekstegers, P., Müller, O.J. et al. (2014). Randomized, controlled trial of ultrasound-assisted catheter-directed thrombolysis for acute intermediate-risk pulmonary embolism. *Circulation* 129 (4): 479–486.

3 Piazza, G., Hohlfelder, B., Jaff, M.R. et al. (2015). A prospective, single-arm, multicenter trial of ultrasound-facilitated, catheter-directed, low-dose fibrinolysis for acute massive and submassive pulmonary embolism: the SEATTLE II study. *J. Am. Coll. Cardiol. Intv.* 8: 1382–1392.

4 Tapson, V.F., Sterling, K., Jones, N. et al. (2018). A randomized trial of the optimum duration of acoustic pulse thrombolysis procedure in acute intermediate-risk pulmonary embolism: the OPTALYSE PE trial. *J. Am. Coll. Cardiol. Intv.* 11: 1401–1410.

5 Tu, T., Toma, C., Tapson, V. et al. (2019). A prospective, single-arm, multicenter trial of catheter-directed mechanical thrombectomy for intermediate-risk acute pulmonary embolism: the FLARE study. *JACC Cardiovasc. Interv.* 12 (9): 859–869.

6 Pasha, A.K., Elder, M.D., Khurram, D. et al. (2014). Successful management of acute massive pulmonary embolism using Angiovac suction catheter technique in a hemodynamically unstable patient. *Cardiovasc. Revasc. Med.* 15 (4): 240–243.

7 D'Ayala, M., Worku, B., Gulkarov, I. et al. (2017). Factors associated with successful thrombus extraction with the AngioVac device: an institutional experience. *Ann. Vasc. Surg.* 38: 242–247.

8 Donaldson, C.W., Baker, J.N., Narayan, R.L. et al. (2015). Thrombectomy using suction filtration and veno-venous bypass: single center experience with a novel device. *Catheter. Cardiovasc. Interv.* 86 (2): E81–E87.

9 Hameed, I., Lau, C., Khan, F.M. et al. (2019). AngioVac for extraction of venous thromboses and endocardial vegetations: a meta-analysis. *J. Card. Surg.* 34 (4): 170–180.

10 Starck, C.T., Eulert-Grehn, J., Kukucka, M. et al. (2018). Managing large lead vegetations in transvenous lead extractions using a percutaneous aspiration technique. *Expert Rev. Med. Devices* 15 (10): 757–761.

11 George, B., Voelkel, A., Kotter, J. et al. (2017). A novel approach to percutaneous removal of large tricuspid valve vegetations using suction filtration and veno-venous bypass: a single center experience. *Catheter. Cardiovasc. Interv.* 90 (6): 1009–1015.

12 Hoeper, M.M. and Granton, J. (2011). Intensive care unit management of patients with severe pulmonary hypertension and right heart failure. *Am. J. Respir. Crit. Care Med.* 184 (10): 1114–1124.

13 Ergan, B., Ergün, R., Çalışkan, T. et al. (2016). Mortality related risk factors in high-risk pulmonary embolism in the ICU. *Can. Respir. J.* 2016.

17

Catheter-Based Therapy for Varicose Veins

Juan Terre and Nelson Chavarria

Division of Cardiology, Albert Einstein College of Medicine-Montefiore Medical Center, Bronx, NY, USA

Introduction

Management of symptomatic chronic venous insufficiency is complex and varies with disease severity [1–4]. In the following series, we describe the use of minimally invasive treatment modalities employed when venous duplex ultrasound imaging confirms the diagnosis and identifies specific segments of venous incompetence [5–7]. Thermal techniques including radiofrequency (RF) ablation and endovenous laser therapy will be discussed, as well as an emerging technology that does not use tumescence or healing elements, mechanico-chemical ablation (MOCA) [8, 9].

Thermal Techniques

Two current methods used to achieve ablation of the great or small saphenous veins involve the use of a RF catheter and an endovenous laser ablation (EVLA) procedure utilizing a laser-fiber catheter, both requiring their own respective generators. The primary difference between the two techniques is the heat source. RF ablation utilizes RF waves to produce steam bubbles and heat to damage the endothelium and denature the collagen matrix of the vein wall. Eventually leading to inflammation and fibrosis. The EVLA method utilizes a laser fiber to directly deliver laser energy to the vein wall causing endothelial damage and subsequent fibrosis. Both modalities require tumescent anesthesia to compress the vein

Endovascular Interventions: A Step-by-Step Approach, First Edition. Edited by Jose M. Wiley, Cristina Sanina, George D. Dangas, and Prakash Krishnan.
© 2023 John Wiley & Sons Ltd. Published 2023 by John Wiley & Sons Ltd.

around the catheter and insulate the surrounding tissue from thermal injury. Below we describe step-by-step techniques of these treatment modalities.

Radiofrequency (RF) Ablation

Step 1. Access to the refluxing superficial vein is first obtained at its lowest point of incompetence under ultrasound guidance (evaluation in short- and long-axis views advised [Figure 17.1]) with a 21G introducer needle and 0.018-in. wire under local anesthesia (1% lidocaine). Utilizing a modified Seldinger technique, a 4 Fr micropuncture sheath is advanced into the vein over the 0.018-in. wire. Techniques employed to increase first puncture success include reverse Trendelenburg positioning, continuous IV hydration, rubber band ligation above the access point, or placement of a warming pad.

(a)   (b)

(c)   (d)

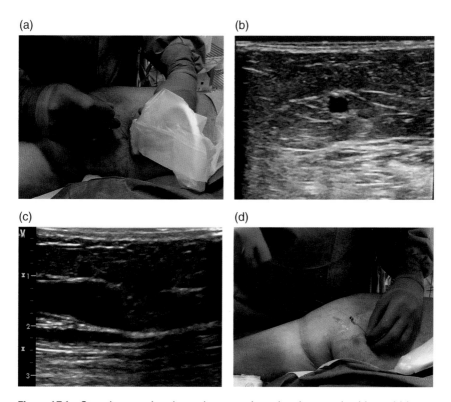

Figure 17.1 Steps in accessing the saphenous vein under ultrasound guidance (a) in short (b) and long-axis views (c), ultrasound guided vein puncture (d).

(a)   (b)   (c)

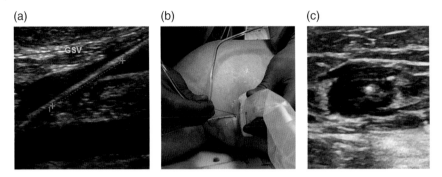

Figure 17.2 Steps in catheter positioning and tumescent anesthesia administration. Catheter advanced and then retracted 2.5 cm from the saphenofemoral junction (a). Injection of tumescent anesthesia under ultrasound guidance (b) creating a "thermal sink" and collapsing the vein around the catheter (c).

Step 2. Once access is secured, the 0.018-in. wire is exchanged for a 0.035-in. guidewire. The 4Fr micropuncture sheath is then exchanged for a 5 Fr introducer sheath. Intraluminal position within the vein is confirmed by aspirating non-pulsatile venous blood and visualization under ultrasound.

Step 3. The RF ablation catheter (Covidien ClosureFast™, Medtronic, MN, USA) is then slowly advanced in the saphenous vein under ultrasound guidance and placed at least 2.5 cm distal of the saphenofemoral junction (Figure 17.2a). Advancing the catheter may sometimes prove difficult when making turns. Pressing the overlying tissue to direct advancement is often helpful.

Step 4. Once the catheter is in place, local tumescent anesthetic solution (450 ml 0.9% normal saline, 35 ml 0.1% lidocaine, and 15 ml 0.8% sodium bicarbonate [10]) is injected under ultrasound guidance in the perivenous space of the saphenous vein (Figure 17.2b,c). Tumescent anesthesia can be administered either manually with serial injections utilizing a 20 cc syringe and 21G needle or with a filtration pump (HK Surgical Klein Infiltration Pump™, HK Surgical Inc., San Clemente, CA, USA), which can deliver high volumes of anesthesia through pressure tubing. Aside from providing anesthesia, tumescent fluid serves to separate the vein from perivenous structures, creating a "thermal sink" to dissipate peak temperatures and compresses the vein to maximize treatment to the endothelial wall.

Step 5. The RF generator is then activated, providing heat energy of 120°C for 20 seconds through the 7 cm copper coil segment of the ablation catheter. Once the treatment cycle is completed after 20 seconds, the catheter is simply withdrawn to the new adjacent venous segment and the generator is activated once again to give another 20 seconds treatment cycle. The steps are repeated in sequence to treat the entire length of the vein.

Step 6. At the end of the procedure, the catheter and sheath are removed. Hemostasis is achieved with manual compression at the site of venous access. Compression bandages and stockings are applied on the treated leg for one to three days to reduce postprocedure bruising and tenderness.

Follow-Up

Patients are encouraged to walk after the procedure. Follow-up protocols vary by institution [11]. In general, patients are encouraged to undergo a repeat venous ultrasound to ensure successful occlusion of the treated vein and confirm the absence of deep venous injury, one to three days postprocedure. The patient is also provided a repeat clinical evaluation in one to three weeks. Long-term therapy comprises encouraging the use of 20–30 compression stockings regularly [12]. The duration of compression stocking therapy is guided by clinical judgment.

Endovenous Laser Ablation (EVLA)

Step 1. Access to the refluxing superficial vein is first obtained at its lowest point of incompetence under ultrasound guidance (long-axis views preferred) with a 21G introducer needle and 0.018 in. wire under local anesthesia (1% lidocaine). Utilizing a modified Seldinger technique, a 4 Fr micropuncture sheath is advanced into the vein over the 0.018-in. wire.

Step 2. Once access is secured, the 0.018-in. wire is exchanged for a 0.035-in. guidewire. Then the 4 Fr micropuncture sheath is exchanged for the long endovenous laser sheath, which is slowly advanced into saphenous vein under ultrasound guidance to the saphenofemoral junction. Intraluminal position of the sheath is confirmed by aspirating nonpulsatile venous blood from the sheath and visualization under ultrasound.

Step 3. Once the sheath is secured in place, a 600 μm laser fiber (Angiodynamics VenaCure EVLT system™, Latham, NY, USA) is advanced through the sheath, to the saphenofemoral junction. While holding the laser fiber in place, the sheath is withdrawn 3 cm to expose the distal bare-tipped laser fiber near the saphenofemoral junction.

Step 4. The sheath and fiber are then pulled back together, so that the tip of the laser fiber is positioned at least 2.5 cm from the saphenofemoral junction.

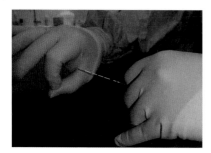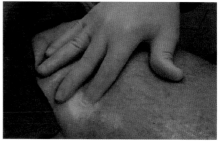

Figure 17.3   EVLA laser tip visualization through the skin with red beam.

Laser-fiber tip positioning is confirmed under ultrasound guidance and with direct visualization of the red beam of the laser fiber through the skin (Figure 17.3).

Step 5. Once the catheter is in place, local tumescent anesthetic solution (450 ml 0.9% normal saline, 35 ml 0.1% lidocaine, and 15 ml 0.8% sodium bicarbonate) is injected under ultrasound guidance in the perivenous space of the saphenous vein.

Step 6. Laser generator is then activated, delivering 12 W of energy to the 810-nm diode laser fiber. While activated, the fiber is slowly withdrawn at an average rate of seven seconds per centimeter to ensure adequate treatment of the venous segments during the slow continuous pull-back.

Step 7. At the end of the procedure, the catheter and sheath are removed. Hemostasis is achieved by manual compression at the site of venous access. Compression bandages and stockings are applied on the treated leg for one to three days to reduce postprocedure bruising and tenderness.

Nonthermal Techniques

Newer nonthermal techniques have emerged in recent years that do not require tumescent anesthesia (reduces number of needle pricks) or exposure to a heating element (reduces potential for pain and nerve injury) [13]. Collectively, they are less traumatic and are associated with fewer local complications with increased patient satisfaction. Cyanoacrylate glue (CAG) ablation and foam sclerotherapy are two forms of noncatheter based, nontumescent, and nonthermal modalities. Here, we will focus on the catheter-based hybrid model, MOCA. It utilizes a special rotating catheter that not only mechanically damages the endothelium inside the vein but also allows for simultaneously infusion a sclerosant solution through the catheter to further injure the vein wall [14]. Free of tumescent and thermal effects, MOCA has emerged as a valid alternative to RF ablation and EVLA catheter-based therapies.

Mechanico-Chemical Ablation (MOCA)

Step 1. Access to the refluxing superficial vein is first obtained at its lowest point of incompetence under ultrasound guidance (long-axis view preferred [15]) with a 21G introducer needle and 0.018 in. wire under local anesthesia (1% lidocaine). Utilizing a modified Seldinger technique, a 4 Fr micropuncture sheath is advanced into the vein over the 0.018-in. wire.

Step 2. Intraluminal positioning of the 4 Fr sheath is confirmed by aspirating nonpulsatile venous blood from the sheath and visualization under ultrasound. Once confirmed the 0.018-in. wire is removed and the catheter (Endovenous ClariVein™, South Jordan, UT, USA) is advanced into the 4 Fr sheath where it is advanced under ultrasound guidance 2.5 cm from saphenofemoral junction. The catheter tip has an angled shape to facilitate directionality during advancement.

Step 3. Tumescent anesthesia is not required for this procedure. Rather, a liquid sclerosant is prepared containing of liquid 1.5% sodium tetradecyl sulfate (2.5 ml of 3% STS and 2.5 ml of 0.9% NS). An alternative to the liquid 1.5% STS, the sclerosant can also be prepared in a foam consistency.

Step 4. Sclerosant foam is prepared by the Tessari method, where a 5 cc syringe containing 1 ml of 1.5% STS and 4 ml of room air is connected to second 5 cc syringe by way of three-way stop cock valve. The syringes are tilted 45° from a flat position and mixed vigorously back and forth 20 times to produce the smallest foam bubbles (Figure 17.4a–c).

Step 5. Once liquid or foam sclerosant is prepared, the catheter is turned on to initiate mechanical damaged to the endothelium, where it rotates 360° at 3500 rpm (high setting). The catheter is then slowly withdrawn at a rate of 2–3 mm/s while simultaneously injecting 0.5 ml of sclerosant (liquid or foam).

Step 6. Once the desired segment is treated, the catheter and 4 Fr micropuncture sheath are withdrawn and hemostasis achieved with manual compression of the venous access site. Compression bandages and stockings are applied on the treated leg for one to three days to reduce postprocedure bruising and tenderness.

(a) (c)

(b)

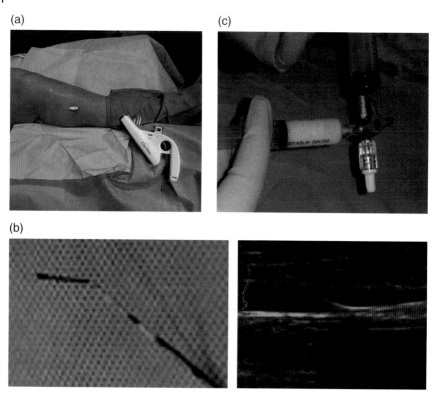

Figure 17.4 The ClariVein device consists of a 9 V battery-motorized handle (a) with infusion catheter that has an angled tip (b). Angled tip allows for steering and directionality (c). Tessari method for sclerosant foam preparation.

Limitations

Despite advances in minimally invasive techniques for saphenous vein ablation, we have observed several aspects of disease location and anatomy that need special consideration when selecting treatment modalities. Thermal techniques involving heat elements typically require 10 cm of subcutaneous tissue above the target vein to prevent skin burns or nerve damage. This is most particularly important when performing below the knee interventions, where nonthermal modalities are often preferred. If a thermal modality is considered, decreasing the voltage and ensuring adequate tumescent anesthesia become critical. Similarly, when encountering aneurysmal vein segments (>10 cm diameter), we have observed better long-term occlusion rates with EVLT versus ClariVein. Firm external compression over the vein segments while delivering treatment cycles is a key for successful outcomes.

Summary

Since the introduction of minimal invasive modalities for the treatment of saphenous vein incompetence, many new techniques have emerged. While most techniques report favorable anatomic success rates, more emphasis is now being placed on the secondary treatment outcomes, such as postprocedural pain, hematoma, quality of life, and return to normal activities. Development of the nontumescent, nonthermal techniques promises to offer many of these advantages. Although proficiency in the "gold standard" techniques of RFA and EVLA is vital, learning these newer techniques such as MOCA can prove effective in achieving excellent results with greater patient satisfaction.

References

1 Davies, A.H. (2019). The seriousness of chronic venous disease: a review of real-world evidence. *Adv. Ther.* 36 (Suppl 1): 5–12. https://doi.org/10.1007/s12325 019 0881-7. Epub 2019 Feb 13. PMID: 30758738.

2 Rabe, E., Guex, J.J., Puskas, A. et al. (2012). Epidemiology of chronic venous disorders in geographically diverse populations: results from the Vein Consult Program. *Int. Angiol.* 31 (2): 105–115.

3 Rice, J.B., Desai, U., Cummings, A.K. et al. (2014). Burden of venous leg ulcers in the United States. *J. Med. Econ.* 17 (5): 347–356. https://doi.org/10.3111/13696998.2014.903258.

4 Labropoulos, N. (2019). How does chronic venous disease progress from the first symptoms to the advanced stages? A review. *Adv Ther.* 36 (Suppl 1): 13–19. https://doi.org/10.1007/s12325-019-0885-3. Epub 2019 Feb 13.PMID: 30758741.

5 Niedzwiecki, G. (2005). Endovenous thermal ablation of the saphenous vein. *Semin. Intervent. Radiol.* 22 (3): 204–208. PMCID: PMC3036276, PMID: 21326694.

6 Bootun, T., Lane, R.A., and Davies, A.H. (2016). A comparison of thermal and non-thermal ablation. *Rev. Vasc. Med.* 4–5: 1–8.

7 Bootun, R., Lane, T.R., and Davies, A.H. (2016). The advent of non-thermal, non-tumescent techniques for treatment of varicose veins. *Phlebology* 31 (1): 5–14. https://doi.org/10.1177/0268355515593186. Epub 2015 Jun 30. PMID: 26130051.

8 Bootun, R., Lane, T.R., Dharmarajah, B. et al. (2016). Intra-procedural pain score in a randomised controlled trial comparing mechanochemical ablation to radiofrequency ablation: the Multicentre Venefit™ versus ClariVein® for varicose veins trial. *Phlebology* 31 (1): 61–65. https://doi.org/10.1177/0268355514551085. Epub 2014 Sep 5. PMID: 25193822.

9 Lane, T., Bootun, R., Dharmarajah, B. et al. (2017). A multi-Centre randomised controlled trial comparing radiofrequency and mechanical occlusion chemically

assisted ablation of varicose veins - final results of the Venefit versus Clarivein for varicose veins trial. *Phlebology* 32 (2): 89–98. https://doi.org/10.1177/0268355516651026. Epub 2016 Jul 9. PMID: 27221810.

10 Wallace, T., Leung, C., Nandhra, S. et al. (2017). Defining the optimum tumescent anaesthesia solution in endovenous laser ablation. *Phlebology* 32 (5): 322–333. https://doi.org/10.1177/0268355516653905. Epub 2016 Jun 15. PMID: 27306991.

11 Carroll, C., Hummel, S., Leaviss, J. et al. (2013). Clinical effectiveness and cost-effectiveness of minimally invasive techniques to manage varicose veins: a systematic review and economic evaluation. *Health Technol. Assess.* 17 (48): i–xvi, 1–141. https://doi.org/10.3310/hta17480. PMID: 24176098; PMCID: PMC4780990.

12 Gloviczki, P., Comerota, A.J., Dalsing, M.C. et al. (2011). The care of patients with varicose veins and associated chronic venous diseases: clinical practice guidelines of the Society for Vascular Surgery and the American Venous Forum. *J. Vasc. Surg.* 53 (Suppl): 2S–48S.

13 Tekin, A.İ., Tuncer, O.N., Memetoğlu, M.E. et al. (2016). Nonthermal, nontumescent endovenous treatment of varicose veins. *Ann. Vasc. Surg.* 36: 231–235. https://doi.org/10.1016/j.avsg.2016.03.005. Epub 2016 Jul 13. PMID: 27421205.

14 Witte, M.E., Zeebregts, C.J., de Borst, G.J. et al. (2017). Mechanochemical endovenous ablation of saphenous veins using the ClariVein: a systematic review. *Phlebology* 32 (10): 649–657. https://doi.org/10.1177/0268355517702068. Epub 2017 Apr 12. PMID: 28403687.

15 Stone, M.B., Moon, C., Sutijono, D., and Blaivas, M. (2010). Needle tip visualization during ultrasound-guided vascular access: short-axis vs long-axis approach. *Am. J. Emerg. Med.* 28 (3): 343–347. [PMID: 20223394].

Index

Endovascular Interventions: A Step-by-Step Approach, First Edition. Edited by Jose M. Wiley,
Cristina Sanina, George D. Dangas, and Prakash Krishnan.
© 2023 John Wiley & Sons Ltd. Published 2023 by John Wiley & Sons Ltd.